The *In Practice* Handbooks

Feline

Practice 2

Edited by E. Boden and M. Melling
Editors, *In Practice*

W. B. Saunders Company Ltd

LONDON   PHILADELPHIA   TORONTO   SYDNEY   TOKYO

W. B. Saunders   24–28 Oval Road
Company Ltd   London NW1 7DX

                      The Curtis Center
                      Independence Square West
                      Philadelphia, PA 19106-3399, USA

                      Harcourt Brace & Company
                      55 Horner Avenue
                      Toronto, Ontario M8Z 4X6, Canada

                      Harcourt Brace & Company, Australia
                      30–52 Smidmore Street
                      Marrickville
                      NSW 2204, Australia

                      Harcourt Brace & Company, Japan
                      Ichibancho Central Building
                      22-1 Ichibancho
                      Chiyoda-ku, Tokyo 102, Japan

A catalogue record for this book is available from the British Library

ISBN 0–7020–2081-8

Typeset by Photo·graphics, Honiton, Devon
Printed and bound in Hong Kong by Dah Hua Printing Press Co., Ltd.

(M) 636. 808 9 B

Feline Pr

The *In Practice* Handbooks Series

Series Editors: Edward Boden and Margaret Melling

Past and present members of *In Practice* Editorial Board

J. Armour (Chairman 1979–1989)

W. M. Allen
I. D. Baker
F. J. Barr
P. B. Clarke
M. J. Clarkson
P. G. G. Darke
A. L. Duncan
J. K. Dunn
G. B. Edwards
S. D. Gunn (Chairman 1990–present)
S. A. Hall
L. B. Jeffcott
B. Martin
H. A. O'Dair
J. Richardson
K. A. Urquhart

Titles in print:
Feline Practice
Canine Practice
Equine Practice
Bovine Practice
Sheep and Goat Practice
Swine Practice
Small Animal Practice
Poultry Practice
Canine Practice 2
Equine Practice 2

Contents

Contributors

S. M. Crispin, University of Bristol, Department of Veterinary Surgery, Langford House, Langford, Bristol BS18 7DU, UK

M. A. Fisher, Brentknoll Veterinary Centre, 152 Bath Road, Worcester, Worcestershire WR5 3EP, UK

N. T. Gorman, The Waltham Centre for Pet Nutrition, Waltham-on-the-Wolds, Melton Mowbray, Leicestershire LE14 4RT, UK

A. L. Hopkins, North Florida Neurology, Department of Veterinary Neurology and Neurosurgery, 1015 South East Lake Lane, Keystone Heights, Florida 32656, USA

C. D. Hopper, Department of Social Medicine, University of Bristol, Canynge Hall, Whiteladies Road, Bristol, Avon BS8 2PR, UK

V. Luis Fuentes, Royal (Dick) School of Veterinary Studies Summerhall Square, Summerhall, Edinburgh EH9 1QH UK

C. T. Mooney, Division of Small Animal Clinical Studies, Department of Veterinary Clinical Studies, University of Glasgow Veterinary School, Bearsden Road, Bearsden, Glasgow G61 1QH, UK

H. A. O'Dair, The Veterinary Hospital, Colwill Road, Estover, Plymouth, Devon PL6 8RP, UK

A. H. Sparkes, Division of Companion Animals, Department of Clinical Veterinary Science, University of Bristol School of

Veterinary Science, Langford House, Langford, Bristol BS18 7DU, UK

R. A. Squires, University of Wisconsin School of Veterinary Medicine, Department of Medical Sciences, 2015 Linden Drive West, Madison, WI 53706–1102, USA

A. H. M. van den Broek, Royal (Dick) School of Veterinary Studies, Summerhall Square, Summerhall, Edinburgh EH9 1QH, UK

A. D. J. Watson, Department of Veterinary Clinical Sciences, The University of Sydney, New South Wales 2006, Australia

Foreword

The importance of continuing professional development for the veterinarian has reinforced the value of the articles presented in *In Practice*. Originally published as a clinical supplement to *The Veterinary Record*, *In Practice* is now firmly established as a prime source of information for the experienced veterinary clinician and student. The articles, each specially commissioned from acknowledged authorities on their subject, are selected by an editorial board representing a broad spectrum of veterinary expertise with the aim of updating existing information or introducing new developments leading to changes in practice.

The convention of casting the articles in the form of 'opinionated reviews' with the emphasis, where appropriate, on differential diagnosis has proved extremely successful and continues to be a distinguishing feature of *In Practice*.

Republishing selected articles, each updated by the author, as *In Practice Handbooks* has proved very popular. For ease of reference, each handbook deals with a particular species or group of related animals. The present volume is one of the second series in what is likely to be a continuing set of *In Practice Handbook* titles.

E. Boden

CHAPTER 1

Differential Diagnosis of Pruritus

HILARY O'DAIR

INTRODUCTION

Cats with pruritus are a common problem in small animal practice. Similar visible lesions may be present for skin diseases of widely differing aetiologies and it is important to explain to an owner, at the outset, that a specific diagnosis cannot usually be reached from a clinical examination alone. Often, the diagnosis requires a careful process of investigation which may take time and effort and the owner must not be given false expectations of an immediate cure. Good communication and owner co-operation are essential.

Pruritus is commonly described as an unpleasant sensation which provokes a desire to scratch. It is a primary cutaneous sensation, resulting from chemical stimulation of nerve endings in the skin by a wide variety of compounds. Proteases, which are released from bacteria, fungi, traumatized epidermal cells, leucocytes and dilated capillaries, are currently considered to be the major mediators of pruritus. However, other mediators such as histamine, serotonin, prostaglandins, peptides and leukotrienes are also considered important. Recently, it has been suggested that histamine may play a more central role in pruritus in the cat (Miller and Scott, 1990).

HISTORY

There are several important facts to ascertain in the history of any cat with skin lesions.

(1) Age and life-style, i.e. multi- or single-cat houseshold, hunting/fighting activity
(2) Diet
(3) Age at onset of pruritus
(4) Nature of the pruritus, i.e. intermittent/seasonal, degree of severity
(5) Presence, type and site of lesions
(6) In-contact animals and humans affected
(7) Evidence of fleas
(8) Previous response to therapy, especially glucocorticoids.

IS ANY HAIR LOSS SELF-INDUCED?

Most cats with skin disorders are presented with a history of hair loss, with or without pruritus. The clinician must decide whether the hair loss is self-induced (pruritic or behavioural) or falling out on its own. The history may be of value here but, as some owners fail to detect their cat pulling out its own hair, it is wise to assume that any hair loss is self-induced, until proven otherwise (see Table 1.1).

Table 1.1 Methods of determining self-induced hair loss.

History	
Direct examination	Short, stubby haircoat
	Normal resistance to epilation
Microscopic examination	Distal hair shafts broken
Faecal examination	Excess amount of hair in stool?
Fit Elizabethan collar	Hair regrowth

PRURITIC OR PSYCHOGENIC?

Having established that the hair loss is self-induced, the clinician must then decide if the cat is truly pruritic or whether the hair pulling is the result of an excessive stereotypic grooming behaviour (psychogenic dermatitis). This latter condition is most commonly reported in the Oriental breeds and the lesions result from excessive licking and chewing, often directed along the dorsum and flanks (Fig. 1.1). A current theory is that the increased grooming leads to a release of endorphins, which then serve a protective function against stress and also reinforce the pathway of stereotypic behaviour (Willemse *et al.*, 1990). This differential diagnosis must always be borne in mind, especially if the history and clinical signs are suggestive. However, because there is no easy way to confirm that a cat is suffering from such a neurosis it is wise to assume at this stage that the cat is actually pruritic. The clinician must then undertake to identify and eliminate all the potential causes of pruritus in the cat before returning to a tentative diagnosis of psychogenic dermatitis (see Tables 1.2–1.4).

The application of an Elizabethan collar for 3–4 weeks may help to determine if hair loss is self-induced, but it can be argued that the use of this alone is inhumane if the cat is suffering from psychogenic dermatitis. The clinician must decide if this method is suitable for an individual case.

Although pruritic conditions can be categorized into several specific groups it is important to remember that an ani-

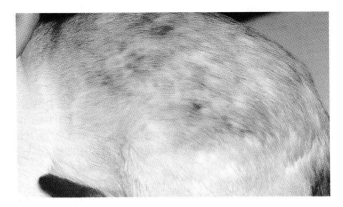

Fig. 1.1
Five-year-old male Siamese with psychogenic alopecia.

Table 1.2 Major differential diagnoses of pruritus in cats can be divided into two main groups.

Hypersensitivity ("allergic") disorders	Ectoparasites
Flea bite	*Ctenocephalides felis*
Atopy	*Cheyletiella* species
Otodectes cynotis	*Otodectes cynotis*
Diet	*Felicola subrostrata*
(Contact)	*Trombicula autumnale* Ticks

Table 1.3 Other differential diagnoses should be considered, but occur less commonly.

Fungal infection, e.g. *Microsporum canis*	*Demodex* species
Bacterial infection	*Sarcoptes* species
Skin neoplasia	Hypereosinophilic
Autoimmune disease	syndrome
Endoparasitic hypersensitivity	Seborrhoeic disorders
Drug eruption	Anal sacculitis

Table 1.4 Clinical signs common to many pruritic disorders in the cat.

Pruritus, especially head and neck

Miliary dermatitis

Alopecia (self-induced) (Fig. 1.4)

Eosinophilic granuloma complex

mal may have more than one condition and that the clinical picture may represent a combination of several different aspects (Fig. 1.2). This combination may include both pruritic and non-pruritic aspects, e.g. psychogenic and hypersensitivity.

Cats with chronic refractory dermatitis should always be evaluated for the presence of the immunosuppressive

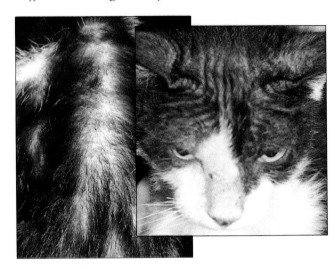

Fig. 1.2
Head and dorsum of a
5-year-old male
domestic shorthair with
Microsporum canis and
dietary hypersensitivity.

viruses, feline immunodeficiency virus (FIV) and feline leukaemia virus (FeLV) (Fig. 1.3).

The following should be considered mandatory in the
approach to a pruritic cat.

(1)   Complete history and physical examination
(2)   Fungal culture and Wood's lamp examination

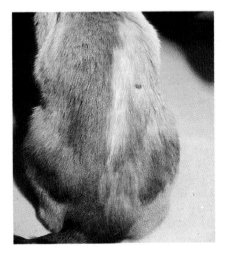

Fig. 1.3
Two-year-old FeLV-positive male Siamese with
hyperaesthesia and self-induced alopecia dorsally.

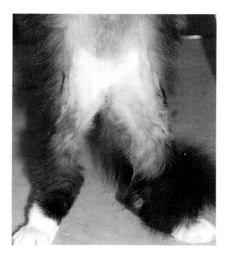

Fig. 1.4
Four-year-old male domestic shorthair with self-induced alopecia (flea bite hypersensitivity) on the ventral abdomen.

(3) Skin scrape(s)
(4) Fine combings
(5) Microscopic examination of affected hair/faeces.

FLEAS

Fleas are the most common ectoparasite of the cat and the single most common cause of pruritus. Non-allergic cats will have few clinical signs of flea infestation, except occasional scratching and licking caused by local irritation from flea bites.

Flea bite hypersensitivity (flea allergic dermatitis) is a frequently seen condition in cats (Table 1.5) which have become sensitized to antigenic components in flea saliva. The immunopathogenesis of the condition is complex. In the dog, both type I and type IV hypersensitivity reactions are documented, while a late-onset IgE reaction and cutaneous basophil hypersensitivity are also thought to be involved. Similar mechanisms are suggested for the feline (Foil, 1986). Clinical signs in affected animals usually consist of papulocrustaceous lesions along the dorsum, in the tailhead region, and around the shoulder and neck region (miliary dermatitis).

Table 1.5 Aids to diagnosis of flea bite hypersensitivity.

Compatible clinical signs
Evidence of fleas or flea excreta
Positive response to intradermal skin testing with flea saliva allergen

In conjunction with
  History
    Evidence of *Dipylidium caninum* infestation (flea is the most common
    intermediate host)
  Evidence of flea infestation of in-contact animals
  Elimination of differential diagnoses
  Positive response to flea control programme

Lesions of the eosinophilic granuloma complex may also be seen (Fig. 1.5). The degree of pruritus can vary from mild to severe. The primary lesions are often masked by secondary self-trauma, and the cat has the ability to cause marked excoriation with both tongue and claws. Increased grooming may remove evidence of fleas and make diagnosis more difficult.

The successful treatment of flea bite disorders is based on the correct management of the flea infestation. Only the adult flea parasitizes the animal, and the remaining 90% of its life cycle is spent in the environment. The major effort at control must be directed at the environment and is the key to success. The following control programme should be considered: restrict access of animals to indoors and to certain rooms only (to keep those flea-free).

In rooms where animal(s) have access:

(1)   Vacuum thoroughly and discard or burn vacuum bag, or steam clean if carpets are deep pile
(2)   Wash all pet bedding, at high temperature if possible
(3)   Use an insecticide spray, strictly according to directions. Those containing a "knock-down" agent and a growth regulator or residual insecticide are the most effective
(4)   Do not vacuum for two weeks after applying spray
(5)   If a growth regulator spray is used, the use of a "knock-down" spray alone, two to three weeks later, will remove any residual adult fleas

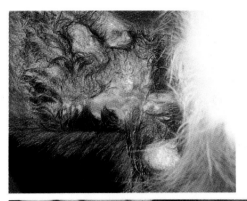

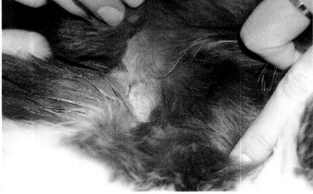

Fig. 1.5
Upper, 6-year-old
male domestic
shorthair with
eosinophilic plaque in
an axilla and lower,
after 10 weeks'
treatment with flea
control and
glucocorticoids.

(6)   This procedure must be repeated on a regular basis, e.g.
every four to six weeks, until control is achieved. The frequency can then be reduced to a maintenance level, e.g. every
four months
(7)   In severe infestations, use of professional pest extermin-
ators may be considered.

INSECTICIDAL TREATMENT OF ALL ANIMALS IN THE HOUSEHOLD

Care must be always be taken in selecting insecticides, because
of the cat's inherent toxic susceptibility, especially to organophosphates. Pyrethroids (synthetic pyrethrins) are the agents of

choice for feline flea control. More recently the phenylpyrazole group (e.g. fipronil) of compounds have proved useful insecticidal agents in the cat. Ease of application, residual efficacy, owner capability and animal temperament are major factors to consider.

Cats rarely tolerate the aerosol noise made by pressurized aerosol sprays so these may be difficult to apply and coat penetration can be poor. Newer pump-action sprays may overcome these problems.

Powders are easier to apply but beware of using excessive amounts. Topical treatments must always be repeated if the cat has got very wet.

The development of synthetic pyrethroids and microencapsulation techniques has improved the efficacy of flea collars but problems of toxicity, contact irritation, duration of activity, and physical trapping of the cat by its collar, must still be borne in mind.

Systemic insecticidal agents, e.g. lufenuron (Program, Ciba Animal Health), may be an option where topical agents cannot be applied. They may be of greater value for in-contact cats, to reduce adult flea numbers, than in a cat with flea bite hypersensitivity. In the latter, the flea saliva (allergen) will already have been injected before the flea is killed. They should be used as part of a long-term flea control programme in multipet households.

Combs may be used by clients who do not wish to use chemicals on their cat. Thorough, repeated combing on a daily basis is required.

Above all, remember that no topical agent will be effective if the environment is still infested.

If an animal has severe flea bite hypersensitivity (see Fig. 1.6) then, despite good owner compliance with flea control regimens, it is likely that some symptomatic therapy will also be required in order to provide reasonable relief from pruritus. The level of therapy can be kept low by constant attention to flea control.

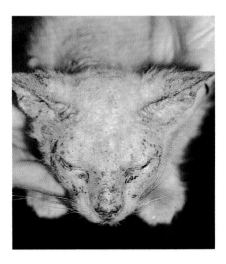

Fig. 1.6
Twelve-year-old male domestic shorthair with severe flea bite hypersensitivity.

OTHER HYPERSENSITIVITY ("ALLERGIC") DISORDERS

ATOPY (INHALANT ALLERGIC DERMATITIS)

Atopy is the term used to describe the hypersensitivity which develops to inhaled allergens such as house dust and pollens. Most animals react to a variety of allergens and signs may be seasonal or continual, depending on the allergen(s) and degree of exposure. In the dog, affected animals have been shown to have a genetic predisposition to form antibodies (IgE, IgG) to these allergens. This is an example of a type I hypersensitivity reaction, with tissue reaction, e.g. mast cell degranulation, occurring within minutes of antigen–antibody combination. Although there is clinicopathological evidence to support the existence of atopy in the cat, neither a reaginic antibody nor genetic (breed) predisposition has yet been isolated.

The clinical manifestations of atopy in the cat are also poorly defined. Most atopic cats develop clinical signs between 6 months and 2 years of age, but signs are variable. Conjunctivitis and rhinitis have also been noted in cats suspected of being atopic. A diagnosis of atopy in a cat would be based upon the following criteria: compatible clinical history and signs; demonstration of skin sensitizing antibody to environmental allergen(s) (positive intradermal skin test); and history of exposure to the allergen(s) coincident with clinical signs.

In practice, the accessibility or economic viability of intra-dermal skin testing may be limited, and the interpretation in the cat still problematic, so a tentative diagnosis of atopy must often rely upon history and signs, and possibly history of exposure to the allergen, supported by thorough elimination of possible differential diagnoses.

Treatment of the atopic cat is based on avoidance of allergen(s), symptomatic therapy, or immunotherapy.

Avoidance is rarely possible but owners may be able to limit the cat's exposure to the allergen(s) and hence reduce signs.

Symptomatic therapy involves the use of anti-inflammatory and non-specific agents to control the clinical signs (see Fig. 1.7). These may be of value when the allergic condition is of short duration, the response to avoidance therapy or immunotherapy is incomplete, or the nature of the hypersensitivity is still obscure (Fig. 1.8). Agents that may be of value in the cat are discussed later in this chapter.

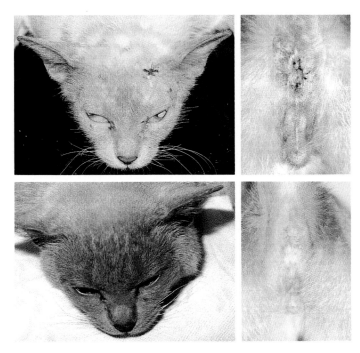

Fig. 1.7 Upper, A 1-year-old male Burmese with atopy of the head and perineum. Lower, after 10 weeks' treatment with glucocorticoids and antihistamines.

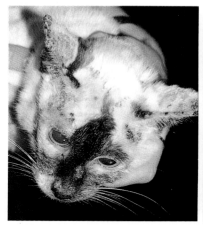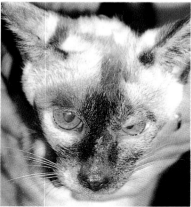

Fig. 1.8 Left, 12-year-old female Siamese with hypersensitivity disorder – the allergen(s) was not identified. Right, after 4 weeks' therapy with glucocorticoids.

Immunotherapy is the term used to describe the attempt to induce tolerance to specific aeroallergens by injecting them at gradually increasing doses on a regular basis. The mechanism by which tolerance develops is still poorly understood. The use of intradermal skin tests and immunotherapy is still comparatively new in the cat, but the documented work to date suggests that both may be of value in the future.

In practice, for the majority of cats with atopic skin disease, symptomatic therapy will still form the basis for management of the condition.

DIETARY

The true incidence of dietary hypersensitivity in the cat is unknown but it should be considered as a possible component in any cat with pruritus. Any age, breed or sex of cat can be affected and any food can be implicated. Clinical signs are variable and non-specific, as in atopy, although facial pruritus may be common (White and Sequoia, 1989; Carlotti *et al.*, 1990; Rosser, 1993). In 10–15% of cases an accompanying gastrointestinal disorder, e.g. recurrent low-grade diarrhoea and / or, vomiting, may be noted. Dietary hypersensitivity is reported to be variably, but often poorly responsive to glucocorticoids.

Diagnosis is by response to dietary elimination. Ideally, a single protein source that has not been fed previously is chosen, e.g. boiled rabbit, with access to fresh water. The addition of boiled rice is optional. No other foods must be fed and it is essential that the owner understands this and is able to comply.

Potential problems include multicat households with shared food bowls, households with indiscriminate feeding by several people, and continued hunting/scavenging. In the feline, palatability and acceptance of the trial diet can also be a problem.

If a dietary hypersensitivity exists, a reduction in pruritus should be seen within the first 2 weeks. However, a diet trial period of at least 30 days is preferable (see Fig. 1.9). Recent studies in dogs with food hypersensitivity suggested that in some individuals a trial period of 8–10 weeks was required (Rosser, 1990). Further work is required to establish definitive recommendations in the cat.

The response should be assessed in the light of other possible concurrent involvement, e.g. seasonal hypersensitivity to pollens. If improvement occurs with the trial diet, the reintroduction of specific dietary elements on a controlled basis should help to confirm or preclude their role in the disorder.

If a cat is to be maintained on a restricted diet long-term then attention must be paid to ensuring adequate levels of dietary taurine, linoleic acid and vitamins. The addition of half

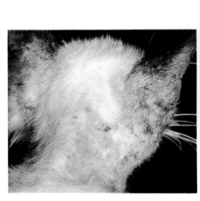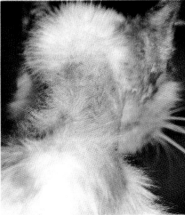

Fig. 1.9 Left, female Birman with dietary hypersensitivity. Right, after 4 weeks on trial diet and antihistamines.

a teaspoon of vegetable oil and dicalcium phosphate, a good vitamin–mineral supplement, and a taurine supplement (the cat's requirement is 15–20 mg/kg daily), should provide a balanced diet.

Commercial hypoallergenic diets for the feline are now becoming available and may be suitable for maintenance in cats with dietary hypersensitivity.

CONTACT

True allergic contact dermatitis (with or without an element of irritant contact dermatitis) is considered to be rare in the cat. However, irritant contact dermatitis, e.g. stepping in an irritant agent, is common. The two conditions are often clinically indistinguishable. The reaction seen in irritant contact dermatitis is usually concentration dependent for any given agent. Lesions can be widespread if the agent has been applied to the whole body, such as a shampoo.

Clinically, lesions generally begin with erythema, swelling and pruritus and progress to chronic thickening, hyperpigmentation and lichenification. In some cases, the contact dermatitis may be secondary to an underlying problem, such as atopy, which has increased the susceptibility of the epidermis to penetration by external agents.

Patch testing, with suspected allergens, is not a practical option in the cat so isolation techniques may be the only way of supporting a tentative diagnosis of contact dermatitis. Removal from the suspect agent or area should last for 7–14 days and, if improvement occurs, provocative re-exposure should help confirm the diagnosis.

OTHER ECTOPARASITES

CHEYLETIELLA SPECIES

Cheyletiella mites are probably more common than previously thought and should always be carefully looked for in combings and skin scrapes (see Fig. 1.10). Clinical signs range from asymptomatic, or mildly scurfy, to extremely pruritic. Treatment with insecticides must include all animals in the household combined with environmental control (mites can survive for up to 10 days off the host).

OTODECTES CYNOTIS

Otodectes cynotis ear mites are common in cats but the degree of clinical disease is variable. Some cats are thought to exhibit a hypersensitivity reaction to the presence of the mites which may induce generalized pruritus.

The mites are large and easily visible microscopically in waxy debris from the ears or, occasionally, in combings/scrapes from other areas of the body.

Treatment involves application of insecticidal drops to the ears. In persistent cases, whole animal and environmental control regimens must also be used.

FELICOLA SUBROSTRATA

Cats are only infested with the biting louse, and kittens are more comonly affected than adults. The adult lice and eggs ("nits") are usually visible to the eye in the haircoat.

Control is relatively straightforward because the life cycle is restricted to the host animal. All animals in the household

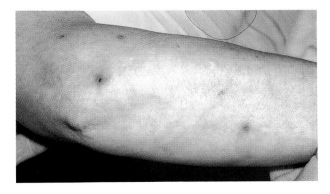

Fig. 1.10
Skin lesions on the arm of an owner of a cat with *Cheyletiella* infestation (photograph, Alan Wright).

should be treated with an insecticidal agent, repeated fort-nightly, until clear.

TROMBICULA AUTUMNALE (HARVEST MITE)

The harvest mite is a free-living mite, the larval form of which parasitizes the cat. It is especially prevalent in the autumn and on chalky soils. The larvae can be seen, often around the feet, chin and ears, as pin-head orange/yellow dots. The best treat-ment is avoidance of infested areas, but if restriction of the cat is impossible then insecticidal sprays or powders may have some effect. Short-term glucocorticoid therapy will relieve pruritus and secondary self-trauma.

SARCOPTES SPECIES/*DEMODEX* SPECIES

These mites have been reported rarely in the feline but, if pres-ent, should be detectable in skin scrapings. Their significance as primary agents is debatable and their presence should prompt the clinician to review the systemic health of the cat, including the possibility of FIV or FeLV involvement.

MICROSPORUM CANIS

The clinical presentation of *Microsporum canis* can vary from asymptomatic to extremely pruritic. Routine examination of a pruritic cat should always include fungal culture.

THERAPEUTIC AGENTS FOR PRURITIC SKIN DISORDERS OF THE CAT

If an ectoparasitic agent is identified, appropriate insecticidal therapy should be instigated.

In hypersensitivity disorders, avoidance of specific allergen(s) should ideally be practised. This may be possible if dietary, con-tact, or flea saliva hypersensitivity are components of the problem. In practice, symptomatic therapy must also be employed in many cases to control the clinical signs.

GLUCOCORTICOIDS

Glucocorticoids are potent and inexpensive anti-inflammatory agents. Although cats appear to be more resistant than dogs to the side-effects of glucocorticoids, great care should still be taken with their use. Oral prednisolone, or methylprednisolone, is the drug of choice and, if therapy is to be long-term, the clinician should always aim for alternate day dosing at the minimum dose required to control clinical signs. An initial dose rate of 1–2 mg/kg/day is suitable for anti-inflammatory use in the cat.

If oral dosing is impractical, injectable depot steroid appears to be well tolerated by the feline and is a viable alternative. Methylprednisolone (Depo-Medrone V, Upjohn) is most suitable, at a dose rate of 4 mg/kg, and ideally no more frequently than once every 8 weeks.

PROGESTOGENS

Although progestogens such as megestrol acetate have been widely used in the treatment of feline skin disorders in the past, the multiplicity and severity of side-effects can weigh heavily against them.

Side-effects of progestogens are:

(1) Profound adrenocortical suppression
(2) Iatrogenic hyperadrenocorticism (Cushing's syndrome)
(3) Polydipsia, polyuria, polyphagia, weight gain
(4) Behavioural changes
(5) Induction of transient or permanent diabetes mellitus
(6) Pyometra
(7) Mammary hyperplasia (see Fig. 1.11) (occasionally leading to neoplasia).

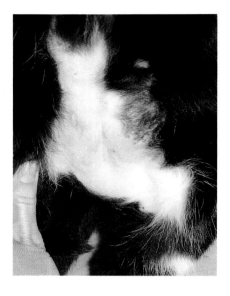

Fig. 1.11
Ventral abdomen of a 10-year-old female domestic
shorthair showing mammary hypertrophy and
ventral alopecia on megestrol acetate therapy.

ANTIHISTAMINES

Antihistamines are not licensed for use in the cat. Dose rates
are not yet standardized and must only be used with the
owner's consent. However, some of the newer antihistamines
appear to be of possible value in the control of pruritus in cats,
with minimal sedative side-effects (see Table 1.6).

Table 1.6 Antihistamines of possible value for pruritus control in the cat.

Generic name	Example	Suggested dosage
Chlorphenarimine maleate	Piriton (Allen & Hanbury)	2 mg bid/tid
Terfenadine	Seldane (Merrell Dow)	10–30 mg bid
Astemizole	Hismanol (Janssen)	2–5 mg bid
Cyproheptadine	Periactin (Merck, Sharp & Dohme)	1–8 mg bid

bid, Twice daily; tid, three times daily.

ESSENTIAL FATTY ACIDS

Essential fatty acids such as Efavit (Efamol) appear to have a significant anti-inflammatory action in certain skin disorders in man and dogs but little work has been done to study their efficacy in cats. No adverse side-effects have been reported and preliminary studies look optimistic (Harvey, 1991, 1993).

ANTIBIOTICS

Cats, unlike dogs, rarely develop pyoderma, except for bite abscesses. If pustules are present, bacterial culture and sensitivity testing from the intact contents should indicate appropriate antibacterial therapy.

TOPICAL AGENTS

Cats are very susceptible to toxicity from some topical agents, such as tars, and there are also practical limitations to their use. In general, the clinician should select the mildest agent possible for the job required. Chlorhexidine (Hibiscrub, Mallinckrodt) is a non-irritant, non-toxic, antibacterial and antifungal agent which does not dry or stain the haircoat. Moisturizing sprays (e.g. Humilac, Virbac) can help cleanse the skin and aid removal of crusts.

OTHER INSECTICIDAL AGENTS

Amitraz dips, at concentrations of 0.025 or 0.05%, are reported to be effective against *Cheyletiella*, *Sarcoptes* and *Demodex* species.

Ivermectin is reported to be effective against *Octodectes cynotis*, *Sarcoptes* species, and *Cheyletiella* (Paradis *et al.*, 1990). A dose rate of 300 µg/kg, by subcutaneous injection, or oral dosing (cattle formulation), repeated twice at 4-week intervals, is appropriate. This should not be used in young kittens.

Note that amitraz and ivermectin are not licensed for use in the cat so must not be used without the owner's consent. No adverse side-effects have been reported in cats.

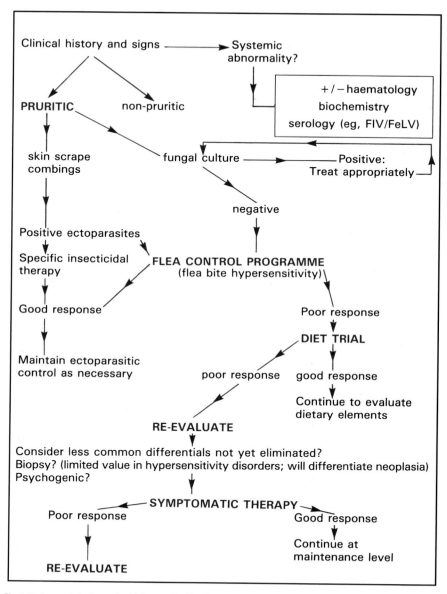

Fig. 1.12 Approach to diagnosis of feline pruritic skin disorders.

SUMMARY

The clinician should make every effort to reach a specific diagnosis in the case of the pruritic cat (see Fig. 1.12). If symptomatic therapy is required, aim for a balanced combination of specific and non-specific therapeutic agents that will provide relief from pruritus, with minimal side-effects.

REFERENCES AND FURTHER READING

August, J. R. (1991) *Consultations in Feline Internal Medicine*. Philadelphia, W. B. Saunders.

Carlotti, D. N., Remy, I. & Prost, C. (1990) Food allergy in dogs and cats: A review and report of 43 cases. *Veterinary Dermatology* **1**, 55–62.

Foil, C. S. (1986) Parasitic dermatoses of the cat. *Solvay Veterinary Dermatology Report* **5**, 2–3.

Halliwell, R. E. W. & Gorman, N. T. (1989) *Veterinary Clinical Immunology*. Philadelphia, W. B. Saunders.

Harvey, R. G. (1991) Management of feline miliary dermatitis by supplementing the diet with essential fatty acids. *Veterinary Record* **128**, 326–329.

Harvey, R. G. (1993) Effect of varying proportions of evening primrose oil and fish oil on cats with crusting dermatosis (miliary dermatitis). *Veterinary Record* **133**, 208–211.

Melman, S. A. & Hutton, P. (1985) Flea control on dogs and cats indoors and in the environment. *Compendium on Continuing Education in the Practicing Veterinarian* **7**, 869–887.

Miller, W. H. & Scott, D. W. (1990) Efficacy of chlorpheniramine maleate for management of pruritus in cats. *Journal of the American Veterinary Medical Association* **197**, 67–70.

Muller, C. H., Kirk, R. W., Scott, D. W., Miller, W. H. & Griffin, C. E. (1995) *Small Animal Dermatology*, 5th edn. Philadelphia, W. B. Saunders.

Paradis, M., Scott, D. W. & Villeneuve, A. (1990) Efficacy of ivermectin against *Cheyletiella blakei* infestation in cats. *Journal of the American Animal Hospital Association* **26**, 125–128.

Reedy, L. M. & Miller, W. H. (1989) *Allergic skin disease of dogs and cats*. Philadelphia, W. B. Saunders.

Rosser, E. J. (1990) Food allergy in the dog: a prospective study of 51 dogs. *ACVD Proceedings*, **47** (Abstr.).

Rosser, E. J. (1993) Food allergy in the cat: a prospective study of 13 cases. *Advances in Veterinary Dermatology* **2**, 1, 2, 33–39.

Schick, M. P. & Schick, R. O. (1986) Understanding and implementing safe and effective flea control. *Journal of the American Animal Hospital Association* **22**, 421–434.

White, S. & Sequoia, D. (1989) Food hypersensitivity in cats: 14 cases 1982–1987. *Journal of the American Veterinary Medical Association* **194**, 692–695.

Willemse, T., Spruijt, B. M. & van Osterwyck, A. (1990) Feline psychogenic alopecia and the role of the opioid system. *Advances in Veterinary Dermatology* **1**, 195–198.

CHAPTER 2

Autoimmune Skin Diseases

ADRI VAN DEN BROEK

INTRODUCTION

Autoimmune skin conditions in cats comprise, in reported order
of incidence, pemphigus foliaceus (most frequent), pemphigus
vulgaris, pemphigus erythematosus, systemic lupus erythematosus and the more recently documented discoid lupus erythematosus (Willemse and Koeman, 1989). All are uncommon.
None appears to have a breed, sex or age predisposition.

Cold agglutinin disease has also been described but is
unlikely to be seen in cats in the UK.

CAUSES

Autoimmune conditions result from immune activity directed
against self-antigens and may be mediated by type II, III or IV
hypersensitivity reactions (Gell and Coombs, 1964).

PEMPHIGUS

The pemphigus group conditions are caused by antibody pro-
duced against self-antigen on the surface of keratinocytes (type
II hypersensitivity) and/or, the cement between keratinocytes.
The ensuing antibody–antigen interaction initiates a process,
sometimes with and sometimes without complement involvement, which results in loss of intercellular cohesion
(acantholysis) and the formation of intraepidermal vesicles
and bullae.

SYSTEMIC LUPUS ERYTHEMATOSUS

Systemic lupus erythematosus (SLE) results from deposition of
immune complexes which provoke complement activity on the
epidermal basement membrane. The immune complexes are
formed by interaction of antibody and self-antigen (type III
hypersensitivity).

Involvement of other systems may arise from deposition of
immune complexes on the basement membrane of other organs,
antibody formation against self-antigen on cells (type II
hypersensitivity) and, although not documented in cats, cell-
mediated activity against self-antigen (type IV hypersensitivity).

The occurrence of these interactions appears to be influenced
by genetic predisposition, activity of T suppressor cells, ultra-
violet light, hormonal factors and, possibly, infectious agents.

DISCOID LUPUS ERYTHEMATOSUS

Discoid lupus erythematosus (DLE), in contrast to SLE, results
from the deposition of immune complexes on the basement
membrane of the skin only.

COLD AGGLUTININ DISEASE

Cold agglutinin disease is caused by autoantibodies active at
low temperatures. These agglutinate red blood cells causing
obstruction of peripheral blood vessels and consequently tissue ischaemia.

CLINICAL SIGNS

PEMPHIGUS

Pemphigus is characterized by the development of bilaterally symmetric intraepidermal vesicles or bullae which are rapidly infiltrated by leucocytes and so form pustules. Unfortunately the thinness of feline epidermis and tendency of cats to rub affected sites combine to promote rapid rupture of vesicles, bullae and pustules. Consequently it is the ensuing signs that are observed. Affected cats usually present with bilaterally symmetric lesions such as oozing erosions or ulcers bordered by epidermal collarettes, erythema, crust and scale formation, localized hair loss and secondary bacterial infection. The drainage lymph nodes may be increased in size. Gentle rubbing at the border of a recently formed erosion or ulcer may result in superficial epidermis peeling off (Nikolsky's sign) and is very suggestive of, though not pathognomonic for, pemphigus. The degree of pain and pruritus associated with the lesions is variable. Similarly the severity of systemic signs, such as depression, anorexia, pyrexia and weight loss, varies.

Pemphigus vulgaris typically involves the mucous membranes of the oral cavity, particularly the hard palate, tongue and pharynx. Ulceration may also occur at the mucocutaneous junction of the lips and nasal philtrum and less frequently elsewhere, i.e. footpads, pinnae, anus, prepuce and vulva. Halitosis may accompany oral lesions.

Pemphigus foliaceus is characterized by crusty scaling lesions of the ears and planum nasale and paronychia with a caseous exudate (Figs 2.1 and 2.2). Mucous membranes are not involved. Crusty, scaling lesions may also occur periorbitally and may extend to involve the body, limbs and face. Marked hyperkeratosis of foot pads may occur and in some cats may be the only observable sign (Fig. 2.3).

Pemphigus erythematosus manifests as crusty scaling lesions usually limited to the face and ears. Paronychia may be present. The mucous membranes are not involved.

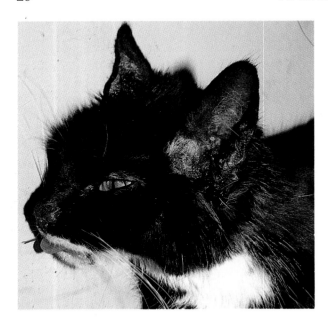

Fig. 2.1
Pemphigus foliaceus:
crusting lesions of the
ears (photograph Mrs J.
Henfrey).

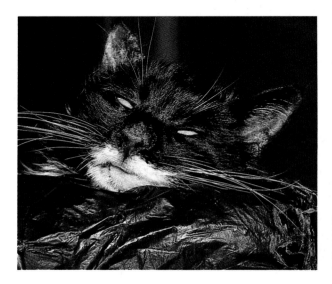

Fig. 2.2
Pemphigus foliaceus:
lesions of the planum
nasale (photograph Mrs
J. Henfrey).

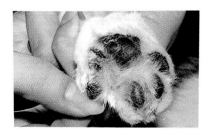

Fig. 2.3
Pemphigus foliaceus: lesions of the limbs (photograph Mrs J. Henfrey).

SYSTEMIC LUPUS ERYTHEMATOSUS

The principal cutaneous manifestation of SLE is a bilaterally symmetric crusty, scaly dermatosis of the face (nasal and peri-orbital areas), ears and paws which may be aggravated by sunlight. Erosions and bullae may occasionally be detected and nasal depigmentation may occur.

Mucocutaneous ulceration of lips and nose may occur but, in contrast to pemphigus vulgaris, oral lesions are uncommon (see Fig. 2.4). Seborrhoea, pruritus and peripheral lymph node enlargement may be prominent signs in some cases. Systemic signs such as depression, anorexia, pyrexia and weight loss are frequently present and, as SLE is a multisystem dis-

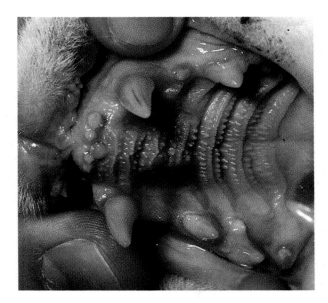

Fig. 2.4
Systemic lupus erythematosus: ulceration of the hard palate (photograph Mrs J. Henfrey).

order, may be accompanied by clinical evidence of anaemia, glomerulonephritis or polyarthritis.

DISCOID LUPUS ERYTHEMATOSUS

Discoid lupus erythematosus presents as a crusty scaly dermatosis which involves the pinnae, body and footpads and may be aggravated by sunlight. Papules, vesicles and erythema may be detected and focal depigmentation of the footpads may occur. The lesions are accompanied by a variable degree of pruritus.

COLD AGGLUTININ DISEASE

Cold agglutinin disease is characterized by erythema, necrosis, sloughing and ulceration of the borders of the pinnae, the nose, the tip of the tail and the paws.

DIAGNOSIS

In cats a bilaterally symmetric crusting/scaling dermatosis of the face and ears with hair loss and secondary bacterial infection, although suggestive of an autoimmune skin disorder, may also accompany other cutaneous disorders. Detection of additional signs, such as cutaneous vesicles/bullae or erosions/ulcers (pemphigus group, occasionally SLE and DLE), and oral erosions or ulcers (pemphigus vulgaris and, less frequently, SLE), digital hyperkeratosis (pemphigus foliaceus), involvement of other body systems (SLE) and necrosis of the extremities of the body (cold agglutinin disease), may be highly suggestive of autoimmune causation and even a particular disease. In these cases the investigation may immediately be directed at confirming the tentative diagnosis. However, in many cases no particular autoimmune marker is observed and a thorough systematic investigation of the possible differential diagnoses is indicated.

Of the differential diagnoses listed in Table 2.1, special note should be taken of drug eruptions. As well as causing type I hypersensitivity reactions (IgE mediated), drugs may induce any one or more of the hypersensitivity reactions (types II, III and IV) involved in the genesis of autoimmune disease. In cats, cimetidine (McEwan *et al.*, 1987) and ampicillin (Mason and Day 1987) have been reported to cause a pemphigus foliaceus-like disease (Figs 2.5 and 2.6). Obviously, if development of the skin lesions was preceded by drug therapy, unless contraindicated, the drug(s) should be withdrawn and if necessary a chemically unrelated drug substituted. The subsequent, spontaneous remission of lesions would support the diagnosis of drug involvement while histopathology and immunofluorescent findings in biopsies of the skin lesions (see below) would indicate the occurrence of drug-induced autoimmunity.

CONFIRMATION OF THE DIAGNOSIS

The Tzanck test (see below) may support a diagnosis of pemphigus but confirmation of pemphigus, SLE and DLE requires demonstration of characteristic histopathological and/or, immunofluorescent changes combined in the case of SLE with detection of a significant antinuclear antibody (ANA) titre or a significant number of lupus erythematosus (LE) cells. All these features are steroid labile, therefore steroid therapy must be discontinued for at least 3 weeks before sampling if reliable results are to be obtained.

PEMPHIGUS

Impression smear (Tzanck test)

In this simple test, direct impression smears of erosions or ulcers are stained and examined using a light microscope. Detection of acantholytic (free-floating) keratinocytes and neutrophils suggests a diagnosis of pemphigus. Haematoxylin and eosin or eosin, thiazine and fast green (Diff Quick, Merz and Dade AG) are suitable stains.

Table 2.1 Differential diagnoses for crusting/scaling dermatoses of the cat and the appropriate investigative procedure(s).

	Investigative procedure(s)
Autoimmune conditions	
Pemphigus vulgaris	Biopsy
Pemphigus foliaceus	Biopsy
Pemphigus erythematosus	Biopsy
Systemic lupus erythematosus	Biopsy, ANA, LE cell preparation
Discoid lupus erythematosus	Biopsy
Cold agglutinin disease	Autoagglutination of blood at 4°C
Hypersensitivity (allergic) conditions	
Atopic disease	Intradermal tests
Food allergy	Dietary restriction
Contact allergy	Environmental restriction
Flea allergic dermatitis	Treatment
Endoparasite hypersensitivity	Treatment
Drug eruption	Drug withdrawal/replacement
Infections/infestations	
Dermatophytosis*	Fungal culture
Bacterial infection*†	Bacterial culture
Parasitic infestations	Skin scrapings
Demodex, Notoëdres*, fleas, lice, Cheyletiella*	
Neoplasia	
Mast cell tumour	Biopsy
Environmental disorders	
Solar dermatitis	Biopsy
Irritant dermatitis	Environmental restriction
Miscellaneous conditions	
Eosinophilic granuloma complex	Biopsy
Relapsing polychondritis of the pinnae	Biopsy
Hypereosinophilic syndrome	Biopsy, circulating eosinophilia
Lichenoid dermatosis	Biopsy
Erythema multiforme	Biopsy
Toxic epidermal necrolysis	Biopsy
Vasculitis	Biopsy

* FeLV, FIV and diabetes mellitus may predispose to fungal and bacterial infections and demodicosis.
† Most bacterial infections are secondary to other conditions.
ANA, Antinuclear antibody; LE, Lupus erythematosus.

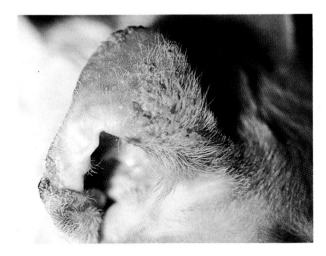

Fig. 2.5
Drug eruption (cimetidine) producing pemphigus foliaceus-like lesions of the ears (reproduced with permission, from McEwan *et al.*, 1987).

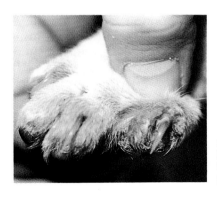

Fig. 2.6
Drug eruption (cimetidine) producing pemphigus foliaceus-like lesions of the feet (reproduced with permission, from McEwan *et al.*, 1987).

Skin biopsy – histopathology and direct immunofluorescent studies

The diagnosis is confirmed in some cases by histopathological examination and in other cases by immunofluorescent studies. Although histopathological changes are considered to be a more reliable indicator for pemphigus, it is advisable to submit samples for both histopathological and direct immunofluorescent studies.

Biopsy sites must be selected carefully. Ideally, the biopsy should include an intact vesicle or bulla and adjacent apparently normal skin. This may necessitate a thorough inspection of the cat every 2 h to detect developing lesions. If this proves impossible several recent erosions or ulcers should be biopsied.

Samples for histopathology should be fixed in 10% formol saline while samples for immunofluorescent studies may be snap-frozen and transported in liquid nitrogen, but are probably more conveniently preserved in Michels Transport Medium which maintains tissue antigenicity for at least 10–14 days. Both samples should be sent to a suitable specialist laboratory. It should be possible to obtain Michels Transport Medium from the specialist laboratory.

The histopathology of pemphigus foliaceus and pemphigus erythematosus is characterized by subcorneal cleft formation and acantholysis. Vesicles and bullae, if present, usually contain acantholytic keratinocytes and neutrophils. Pemphigus vulgaris is distinguished by suprabasilar cleft formation which leaves the basal cells standing like a row of tombstones on the basement membrane.

In all these conditions direct immunofluorescent studies reveal a chicken-mesh pattern of fluorescence, demonstrating the deposition of immunoglobulin (usually IgG) in intercellular spaces throughout the epidermis. In cases of pemphigus erythematosus an additional linear "lupus band" of immunofluorescence occurs at the dermoepidermal junction.

Blood sample – ANA titre

A positive ANA titre may be detected in cases of pemphigus erythematosus. The test requires 1–2 ml of serum, which is submitted to a suitable laboratory.

SYSTEMIC LUPUS ERYTHEMATOSUS

Confirming a tentative diagnosis of SLE is not straightforward and a full discussion of the criteria involved is beyond the scope of this chapter. Briefly, two sets of criteria have been proposed for the diagnosis of SLE in dogs (Bennett, 1987; Halliwell and Gorman, 1989) and both may provide a suitable basis for its diagnosis in cats. In both schemes serological evidence, a positive ANA titre (Bennett, 1987), or positive LE cell preparation (Halliwell and Gorman, 1989) is essential to the diagnosis. Its absence rules out SLE. In addition to serological evidence a combination of clinical, laboratory and immunopathological evidence compatible with a diagnosis of SLE and indicating the involvement of two or more body systems is required. Only evidence from skin biopsies and serology will be dealt with in this chapter.

Blood sample – ANA titre, LE cell preparations

The LE cell preparation requires 5–10 ml of clotted or heparinized blood which needs to be presented to a suitable laboratory within hours of collection.

The ANA test is very sensitive but not specific for SLE while the LE cell preparation is less sensitive but more specific than the ANA test.

Skin biopsy – histopathology and immunofluorescent studies

In suspected SLE, as in pemphigus, skin biopsies should be submitted for both histopathology and immunofluorescent studies.

For histopathology recent and inflamed lesions should be biopsied and fixed in 10% formol saline. In contrast, lesions selected for immunofluorescent studies should be at least 3 weeks old and preferably from an area exposed to sunlight. The lesion and adjacent normal skin should be biopsied and transported in liquid nitrogen or Michels Transport Medium.

Histopathology findings associated with SLE are hydropic or lichenoid change of the basal cell layer (interface dermatitis), thickening of the basement membrane zone, mononuclear cell infiltration around hair follicles and epitrichial (apocrine) and sebaceous glands. Occasionally, evidence of subcorneal vesicles or bullae is present.

Direct immunofluorescent studies demonstrate a "lupus band" of immunoglobulin at the basement membrane zone in the area of the lesion and extending into adjacent normal skin.

DISCOID LUPUS ERYTHEMATOSUS

Skin biopsy – histopathology and immunofluorescent studies

The biopsies should be selected and transported as indicated for SLE. The histopathology of DLE is similar to that of SLE but includes the presence of Civatte (colloid) bodies in the basal cell layer.

As with SLE, direct immunofluorescence reveals a lupus band of immunoglobulin at the basement membrane zone. This should not extend into the adjacent normal skin.

COLD AGGLUTININ DISEASE

Diagnosis is readily confirmed by microscopic observation of red blood cell agglutination when blood samples containing anticoagulant are cooled to −4°C and its reversal when they are warmed to 37°C.

TREATMENT

Treatment of autoimmune skin disorders in cats is routinely initiated by administering a high oral dose of prednisolone (2–3 mg/kg twice daily). Once remission is achieved this dose is gradually reduced to the minimum alternate day dose required to maintain remission. In cases failing to respond, this regimen may be modified by combining prednisolone with other drugs such as azathioprine, sodium aurothioglucose or cyclophosphamide.

Azathioprine has been combined successfully with prednisolone to induce remission in cases of pemphigus foliaceus (Caciolo *et al.*, 1984). However, it is potentially hepatotoxic and may cause bone marrow suppression. In the series of cases referred to, half the cats developed leucopenia after 8.25 doses (1.1 mg every 48 h). It is essential therefore to restrict its use to the induction phase and monitor liver function and routine haematology weekly.

Sodium aurothioglucose may also be combined successfully with prednisolone in the treatment of pemphigus and SLE. Two test doses (1 mg per cat) of sodium aurothioglucose or aurothio-malate are given by intramuscular injection at an interval of 7 days in order to detect any idiosyncratic drug reaction. If none occurs further intramuscular injections of 1 mg/kg are given weekly until clinical improvement is evident, usually 6–12 weeks, and then given monthly.

Cyclophosphamide given orally (50 mg/m^2.day) may be used in cases of SLE refractory to prednisolone. Because it depresses bone marrow activity, routine haematology and platelet numbers should be monitored weekly.

Avoidance of direct sunlight and use of sun screens may be of benefit in cases of pemphigus erythematosus and systemic discoid lupus erythematosus.

ACKNOWLEDGEMENTS

The author would like to thank Mrs J. Henfrey for the photographs of cats with pemphigus foliaceus and systemic lupus erythematosus, Mr N. McEwan for the photographs of the cat with pemphigus foliaceus-like lesions and Mrs L. Reid for typing the manuscript.

REFERENCES

Bennett, D. (1987) Canine systemic lupus erythematosus. *Veterinary Annual* (eds. Grunsell, C. S. G., Hill, F. W. G. and Raw, M. E.), 27th Issue, pp. 350–356. Oxford, Blackwell Science.

Caciolo, P. L., Nesbitt, C. H. & Hurvitz, A. I. (1984) Pemphigus foliaceous in eight cats and results of induction therapy using azathioprine. *Journal of American Animal Hospital Association* 20, 571–577.

Gell, P. G. H. & Coombs, R. R. A. (1964) *Clinical Aspects of Immunology.* Philadelphia, F. A. Davis.

Halliwell, R. E. W. & Gorman, N. T. (1989) *Veterinary Clinical Immunology.* (eds. Halliwell, R. E. W. and Gorman, N. T.). Philadelphia, W. B. Saunders

Mason, K. V. & Day, M. J. (1987) A pemphigus foliaceus-like eruption associated with the use of ampicillin in a cat. *Australian Veterinary Journal* 64, 223–224.

McEwan, M. A., McNeil, P. E., Kirkham, D. & Sullivan, M. (1987) Drug eruption in a cat resembling pemphigus foliaceus. *Journal of Small Animal Practice* 28, 713–720.

Willemse, T. & Koeman, S. P. (1989) Discoid lupus erythematosus in cats. *Veterinary Dermatology* **1**, 19–24.

APPENDIX

The immunological investigations referred to in this article are carried out by the institutes/companies listed in Table 2.2.

Table 2.2 Immunological investigation services.

	Coombs' test	ANA	Immunofluorescent studies
Bloxham Laboratories, Devon	✓	✓	—
Department of Pathology and Microbiology, Bristol School of Veterinary Science	✓	✓	✓
Department of Clinical Veterinary Medicine, Cambridge University	✓	✓	—
Department of Veterinary Pathology, Glasgow University	✓	✓	✓
Department of Pathology, Royal (Dick) School of Veterinary Studies, Edinburgh	—	✓	✓

ANA, Antinuclear antibody.

CHAPTER 3

Systemic Antimicrobial Drug Therapy

A. D. J. WATSON

INTRODUCTION

Drugs are often used in feline practice to treat known or suspected microbial infections. Systemic administration is indicated in most instances, except for a few conditions in which topical application might be adequate, such as superficial infections of the eye or skin or in otitis externa. This situation resembles that in other species, although there are several factors which create special difficulties with systemic drug therapy in cats.

SPECIAL CONSIDERATIONS

Particular problems affecting feline drug therapy relate to the peculiarities of drug metabolism in cats, the limited data on drug efficacy and safety in this species, lack of suitable formulations or dosage units, and problems in drug administration.

PHARMACOLOGY AND TOXICOLOGY

Clinical pharmacology studies in cats can be difficult because, as Brancker (1962) remarked of cats, "the temperament is mercurial, the muscular strength fantastic and the speed in response to stimuli is spectacular". Thus, experimental data supporting safe and effective drug use in feline patients are limited. It is often necessary to extrapolate drug doses and frequencies from other species, for which purpose canine data may be most useful. However, cats are relatively deficient in their ability to conjugate drugs with glucuronic acid. This is an important process which produces less toxic, more water-soluble metabolites for excretion. Where glucuronidation is known to be a major method of inactivation of a potentially toxic drug, such as chloramphenicol, accumulation of drug *in vivo* can be avoided by using lower doses or lengthening the interval between them. However, care is needed when extrapolating data on new or unfamiliar drugs from other species to cats.

FORMULATIONS

The problems of solid dosage units (tablets, capsules) which contain too much drug for the average cat and injectable preparations too concentrated to permit accurate dosing are familiar to all feline practitioners. We are sometimes forced to prescribe larger than desired doses at less frequent than ideal intervals, while hoping that safety and efficacy will not be compromised. For drugs which are bactericidal and relatively non-toxic, like penicillins and cephalosporins, problems are unlikely. However, there may be difficulties with agents that are bacteriostatic (e.g. chloramphenicol, tetracyclines) or potentially toxic (aminoglycosides). Unfortunately, these problems will continue unless manufacturers can be convinced of the need to develop more appropriate formulations for small animal patients. In the meantime it may sometimes be necessary to divide tablets accurately for owners, repackage medications in gelatin capsules, or make precise dilutions of liquid formulations.

DIFFICULTIES IN DOSING

The temperament and physical characteristics of cats make some patients a nightmare to dose, even for skilled operators. Although the compliance rate for drug therapies in cats has not been examined in detail, it would not be surprising to find a large discrepancy between what veterinarians recommend and what owners achieve. Consequently, it is imperative to simplify treatments wherever possible, avoiding unnecessary medications and selecting routes and frequencies that the owner can manage and the cat will tolerate. Otherwise the likely outcome is an angry cat with a dispirited, damaged owner.

ORAL ADMINISTRATION

Dosage by the oral route is adequate in most infections and, with rare exceptions, is the only satisfactory method for home treatment. A struggle over oral medication can be counter-productive and dangerous, however, because of the risk of aspiration pneumonia, especially with oily medicines. There are undoubtedly many ways to handle the cat which is difficult to dose with tablets and capsules; the author prefers to use haemo-stats for this purpose. One hand grasps the cat's scruff and an ear, the head is bent up and back on the neck until the mandible sags, then the tablet or capsule held loosely in the haemostat's jaws is pushed quickly down between tongue and palate to the pharynx, whereupon the drug is released and the instrument withdrawn. An alternative is to hold the cat's head similarly, slide a small teaspoon bearing the tablet into the oropharynx, then tilt the spoon to deposit the drug. These techniques are quick, easy and safe when performed properly. Some owners find it easier to use liquid formulations. These need to be reasonably palatable for cats if a struggle is to be avoided. A plastic dropper can be used, introduced into the side of the mouth in the space behind a canine tooth. To minimize risks of aspiration, the head should be kept steady and almost level, not forced up or back, and the volume given each time should not exceed that which the cat can swallow with ease (Holzworth and Stein, 1987). Naso-oesophageal or orogastric intubation offer alternatives for in-hospital use.

Administration of liquids, powders or crushed tablets mixed in food may be possible, although many cats reject medicated food. Occasionally, they can be fooled into swallowing morsels of a favourite food containing a tablet or capsule, if first offered unmedicated pieces. In all cases, the potential effect of ingesta on drug bioavailability should be considered (see Table 3.1).

PARENTERAL ADMINISTRATION

Injections are often unnecessary for antimicrobial therapy in cats, and some clinicians rarely use them. However, parenteral administration can be valuable to initiate treatment in severe infections where rapid systemic drug availability is important. Other indications include fractious, unconscious or vomiting patients, or those with mouth pain.

The intravenous route should be used if maximum plasma antibiotic concentrations are desired immediately after dosing, as with life-threatening infections. Intravenous use might also be preferable in shocked or hypotensive patients, as poor peripheral perfusion may impede drug absorption from other sites.

Intramuscular or subcutaneous administration is usually safer, and is satisfactory in less demanding circumstances. These routes give similar bioavailability with most preparations tested, although subcutaneous injection is easier and generally causes less pain. Many veterinarians have found that formu-

Table 3.1 Suggested oral administration in relation to feeding.

Better when fasting	Better with food	No restriction needed
Cephalosporins	Chloramphenicol	Chloramphenicol
Erythromycin free base	palmitate	tablets and capsules
Erythromycin stearate	Doxycycline	Erythromycin-coated
Lincomycin	Erythromycin esters	formulations
Most penicillins	Griseofulvin	Fluoroquinolones
Most sulphonamides	Ketoconazole	
Most tetracyclines	Metronidazole	
	Nitrofurantoin	

Data extrapolated from human studies, except for penicillins (from dogs) and chloramphenicol (from cats). "Fasting" means no food for 1–2 h before and 1–2 h after dosing.

lations recommended for intramuscular use in other species generally can be administered effectively to cats by subcutaneous injection (Holzworth and Stein, 1987). However, it would be prudent to test unfamiliar preparations in a few animals prior to clinical use by this route, to check for possible reactions at the injection site.

Should intramuscular injection be deemed necessary, consider using the lumbar longissimus muscle. The site is the lumbar region midway between the iliac crest and last rib, and half-way between the dorsal spinous processes and lateral border of the muscle. Injection here might be partly intramuscular and partly intermuscular, but bioavailability is likely to be as for other intramuscular and subcutaneous injection sites. Injections in this region are usually well tolerated and avoid the risk of sciatic nerve damage.

DRUG SELECTION

The principles governing selection of appropriate antibacterial drugs for use in cats are the same as for other species. Of prime importance is an adequate clinical assessment, which should identify the system or systems involved and the pathogens likely to be responsible. Although increased rectal temperature is compatible with bacterial infection, it is certainly not diagnostic; elevations occur in various other pathological conditions (viral infections, neoplasms, drug reactions, immune-mediated disorders and other non-septic inflammations) and physiological states (exercise, excitement, high ambient temperature). Likewise, leucocytosis is not pathognomonic for infection and can occur with non-septic inflammatory processes, neoplasms, trauma, excitement, stress, and glucocorticoid administration. When a bacterial infection is suspected, identification of the likely pathogen(s) can be facilitated by examination of smears of exudates or aspirates from the infected site, stained by Gram stain and/or, a Romanovsky method (Giemsa, Diff-Quik). *In vitro* culture and susceptibility testing more closely approach the ideal, but are often not feasible because of added costs and lack of facilities. However, in very serious, recurrent or non-responding infections, cost–benefit analysis

Table 3.2 Antimicrobial drug selection for some feline infections.*

Diagnosis	Common infecting organisms	Comments	Suggested drugs	Alternative drugs
Skin and subcutis sites				
Impetigo	β-haemolytic streptococci	Systemic drugs often unnecessary, use local cleansing, antiseptics	Penicillin G or V	
Folliculitis, furunculosis, cellulitis	β-haemolytic streptococci, *Staphylococcus* species	Prolonged therapy (6–9 w) may be needed for deep or recurrent lesions	Penicillin G or V or (for staphs) lincomycin	Amoxycillin-clavulanate
Dermatomycosis	*Microsporum canis*	Use topical and environmental measures as well as or instead of systemic therapy	Griseofulvin	Ketoconazole
Feline "leprosy"	*Mycobacterium lepraemurium*	Surgical removal preferred	Clofazimine	Rifampicin, dapsone
Atypical mycobacterial granuloma	*M. fortuitum*, *M. chelonei*, *M. xenopi*, *M. smegmatis*	Surgical excision and debridement needed. Identification and susceptibility test advised	Fluoroquinolone	Aminoglycosides, tetracyclines, chloramphenicol, erythromycin
Cryptococcal nodules	*Cryptococcus neoformans*		Flucanazole	Itraconazole, ketoconazole plus flucytosine
Cat fight abscess	*Pasteurella multocida*, *Actinomyces* species, various anaerobes	Use hot packs and surgical drainage as necessary	Penicillin G or V	Chloramphenicol, lincomycin, clindamycin

Alimentary and abdominal sites

			First choice	Alternative
Periodontitis and gingivitis	Mixed facultatives and anaerobes	Remove calculus, improve dental hygiene. If severe, consider antibiotic prior to dentistry	Penicillin G or V, amoxycillin	Metronidazole, amoxycillin-clavulanate
Acute ulcerative stomatitis	Various resident bacteria including anaerobes	Infection primary or secondary: seek underlying cause. Remove calculus. Local and supportive treatment important	Penicillin G or V	Metronidazole
Chronic proliferative stomatitis	Infection secondary	Antimicrobials non-curative. Biopsy. Local treatment. Consider systemic glucocorticoid		Metronidazole, penicillins
Bacterial enteritis	*Campylobacter jejuni*	Isolation of doubtful significance. Treatment may be unwarranted	Erythromycin	Chloramphenicol, tetracyclines
	Escherichia coli	As for *Campylobacter*	Chloramphenicol	Aminoglycosides
	Salmonella typhimurium	Uncommon, mainly immunosuppressed cat, or kittens poorly maintained. Use antibiotic only if systemically ill. Treatment may increase persistent carrier rate	Sulphonamide-trimethoprim	Chloramphenicol
Giardiasis	*Giardia* species	Rare in cats	Metronidazole	Tinidazole, furazolidone, quinacrine

Table 3.2 Continued

Diagnosis	Common infecting organisms	Comments	Suggested drugs	Alternative drugs
Coccidiosis	Isospora species, others	Presence of coccidia may be unrelated to cause of diarrhoea	Sulphonamides, sulphoamide-trimethoprim	Furazolidone
Parvoviral enteritis (panleukopenia, feline infectious enteritis)	Secondary bacteria, especially anaerobes	Treat parenterally. Fluid therapy, nursing and supportive care essential	Penicillin G	Ampicillin, or amoxycillin, possibly with gentamicin
Cholecystitis/chol-angio-hepatitis	Coliforms		Amoxycillin-clavulanate	Chloramphenicol
Liver failure, hepatic encephalopathy	Normal intestinal flora	Use low protein diet, lactulose, administer drugs orally	Metronidazole	Amoxycillin-clavulanate
Intra-abdominal sepsis (bacterial peritonitis, abscessation)	Mixed anaerobes and coliforms	Surgery may be necessary. Culture and susceptibility test advisable	Gentamicin plus either clindamycin, doxycycline or metronidazole	Amoxycillin-clavulanate, chloramphenicol
Respiratory and thoracic sites				
Acute viral upper respiratory tract infection	Secondary bacteria: *Staphylococcus* species, β-haemolytic streptococci, *Pasteurella multocida*	Nursing and supportive care essential	Penicillin G or V	Amoxycillin, ampicillin, erythromycin, tylosin

Condition	Organisms	Comments	First choice	Alternative
Chronic rhinitis-sinusitis	As above, plus anaerobes	Intermittent treatment may control, but not cure, the condition	Penicillin V	Amoxycillin, ampicillin, sulphonamide–trimethoprim, chloramphenicol
Cryptococcal rhinitis-sinusitis	*Cryptococcus neoformans*		Fluconazole	Ketoconazole plus flucytosine, itraconazole, amphotericin B
Aspiration pneumonia	Anaerobes	Treat on suspicion if aspiration occurs	Amoxycillin-clavulanate, penicillin G	Chloramphenicol
Other bacterial pneumonia	Various anaerobes, *Pasteurella multocida*, other Gram-negative bacteria, *Actinomyces* species	Culture and susceptibility testing of transtracheal aspirate or bronchial wash recommended	Amoxycillin-clavulanate	Chloramphenicol, sulphonamide–trimethoprim
Pyothorax	Various anaerobes, *Pasteurella multocida*, *Actinomyces* species	Chest drainage and local therapy also needed. Gram-stained smears should be examined	Penicillin G, other penicillins	Chloramphenicol, metronidazole
Miscellaneous Bacterial lower urinary infection	*E. coli*, *Streptococcus* species, *Staphylococcus* species, *Proteus* species	May be secondary to idiopathic nonseptic feline urological syndrome. Antibacterial inappropriate unless bacteriuria present	Amoxycillin-clavulanate	Chloramphenicol, sulphonamide–trimethoprim

Table 3.2 Continued

Diagnosis	Common infecting organisms	Comments	Suggested drugs	Alternative drugs
Feline infectious anaemia	*Haemobartonella felis*	Some cases secondary to immunosuppressive viruses. Consider prednisolone as well as antimicrobial if primary	Tetracyclines	Chloramphenicol
Osteomyelitis	*Staphylococcus* species, *Streptococcus* species	Surgical intervention, susceptibility test advised. Gram-negative bacteria, anaerobes present sometimes	Amoxycillin-clavulanate	Cloxacillin
Toxoplasmosis	*Toxoplasma gondii*		Clindamycin	Sulphonamide plus pyrimethamine
Meningitis	*Pasteurella multocida*, *Staphylococcus* species, *Streptococcus* species	Isolation and susceptibility test recommended	Penicillin G, amoxycillin-clavulanate	Chloramphenicol
Cryptococcus neoformans	Guarded prognosis	Fluconazole	Itraconazole, ketoconazole plus flucytosine	

* These suggestions are based on the author's personal experience, discussion with colleagues and review of the literature. The author finds that the most useful agents generally are the penicillin group and sulphonamide–trimethoprim, with aminoglycosides, lincosamides and metronidazole useful in selected cases. He considers that chloramphenicol is a useful second choice for some infections, but acknowledges that others may favour an alternative because of human health concerns. Some clinicians prefer cephalosporins or quinolones for certain of the infections listed. While these agents are of undoubted value in individual cases, it is his prejudice that there are few indications for the

will favour further microbiological investigation rather than treatment solely on a best-guess basis.

In practice, drug selection is often based on knowledge of the site of infection and the pathogens most frequently implicated, coupled with the likely susceptibility of the infecting organisms (see Table 3.2).

Where several drugs are likely to be effective against the pathogen, possible costs, routes and toxic potential will influence the final selection of the drug to be used. Drug selection may need to be modified in renal failure, liver failure, pregnancy or in neonates (see Table 3.3). If all other things are equal, the antimicrobial with narrowest spectrum should be chosen, to reduce the selection pressure for resistance exerted by broad-spectrum agents.

Conventional dosage regimens for commonly used drugs are presented in Table 3.4. Some flexibility in treatment is appropriate as the optimum regimen will vary with the infection, depending on the susceptibility of the organism, the extent of drug penetration into infected tissues and the integrity of the host's defence mechanisms.

Table 3.3 Antimicrobial drugs which are potentially hazardous in renal failure, liver failure, pregnancy or in neonates.

Renal failure	Liver failure	Pregnancy	Neonates
Aminoglycosides	Chloramphenicol	Aminoglycosides	Aminoglycosides
Amphotericin B	Clindamycin	Amphotericin B	Chloramphenicol
Carbenicillin	Erythromycin	Chloramphenicol	Fluoroquinolones
Cephaloridine	estolate	Flucytosine	Nalidixic acid
Chloramphenicol	Lincomycin	Fluoroquinolones	Nitrofurantoin
Flucytosine	Oxacillin	Griseofulvin	Polymyxins
Fluoroquinolones	Tetracyclines	Ketoconazole	Sulphonamides
Nalidixic acid		Metronidazole	Tetracyclines
Nitrofurantoin		Nitrofurantoin	Trimethoprim
Polymyxins		Polymyxins	
Tetracyclines		Sulphonamides	
(except		(long acting)	
doxycycline)		Tetracyclines	
		Trimethoprim	

Table 3.4 Conventional dosage regimens for antimicrobial drugs in cats.

Drugs	Route of administration	Dose mg/kg (except as indicated)	Hours between doses
Aminoglycosides			
Amikacin	iv,im,sc	5–10	8–12
Dihydrostreptomycin	po	10–20	6
	im,sc	10	12
Gentamicin	iv,im,sc	2–4	8–12
Kanamycin	po	10–12	6
	iv,im,sc	5–10	8–12
Neomycin	po	10–20	6
Streptomycin	po	20	6
	im,sc	10	12
Tobramycin	iv,im,sc	1–2	8

Notes: Bactericidal, active against certain Gram-negative facultative bacteria, some mycobacteria, some mycoplasma. Ineffective against anaerobes. Poorly absorbed from the gut. Generally penetrate tissues and body fluids poorly. Excreted unchanged in urine. Potential toxicity: vestibular damage, hearing loss, neuromuscular block, renal damage. Avoid prolonged systemic use, ensure adequate hydration. Nephrotoxicity indicated by increased urine volume, protein and casts, reduced specific gravity, and azotaemia. Recent studies suggest administration of total daily dose in one bolus rather than split doses may reduce toxic risk without compromising efficacy.

Antifungals			
Amphotericin B	iv	0.2–0.5	48

Notes: Nephrotoxic. Give by iv infusion. Consult texts.

Flucytosine	po	100	12–24

Notes: Combine with ketoconazole or amphotericin B. Side effects: vomiting, diarrhoea, leucopenia, thrombocytopenia.

Fluconazole	po	50 mg per cat	8–12

Notes: Liver enzymes may increase. Inappetence in some cats.

Griseofulvin	po	25–60	12

Notes: Teratogenic. May cause gut upsets, anaemia, leucopenia, pruritus, ataxia.

Ketoconazole	po	10	12–24

Notes: Use alone for dermatomycosis. Combine with flucytosine for cryptococcosis. May cause anorexia, depression, diarrhoea, fever. Avoid in pregnancy (embryotoxic, teratogenic).

Table 3.4 Continued

Drugs	Route of administration	Dose mg/kg (except as indicated)	Hours between doses
Cephalosporins			
Cephadroxil	po	20	12–24
Cephalexin	po	20–30	8
Cephalothin	iv,im,sc	20–35	6–8
Cephapirin	iv,im,sc	30	6
Cephradine	po,iv,im	20	6

Notes: Bactericidal, non-toxic, excreted in urine. Several first generation agents are listed. These are generally resistant to staphylococcal penicillinase and active against many Gram-positive and some Gram-negative bacteria. Possible uses against penicillin-resistant staphylococci, anaerobes and some urinary or soft tissue infections caused by Gram-negative facultative bacteria. Later cephalosporins have enhanced activity against some Gram-negative pathogens but cost may be prohibitive.

Macrolides and lincosamides			
Clindamycin	po,iv,im	10–25	8–12
Erythromycin	po	10–20	8–12
Lincomycin	po	10–20	8–12
	iv,im	10–20	12–24
Tylosin	po	10	8
	iv,im	5–10	12

Notes: Bacteriostatic, similar spectra to penicillin G. Macrolides (erythromycin, tylosin) also active against chlamydia, rickettsia and mycoplasma, and lincosamides (lincomycin, clindamycin) against mycoplasma. Clindamycin useful (at higher dose) in toxoplasmosis. Excreted mainly in bile. Some also in urine. Cause mild gastrointestinal upsets (vomiting, diarrhoea) in some patients.

Penicillins, narrow spectrum
Notes: Bactericidal, used mainly against Gram-positive facultative bacteria, anaerobes and *Pasteurella multocida*

Penicillin G, Na or K	iv,im,sc	20,000–40,000 U/kg	4–6

Notes: Provides rapid, high concentrations.

Penicillin G, procaine	im,sc	20,000 U/kg	12–24

Notes: Slower absorption, more prolonged effect.

Table 3.4 Continued

Drugs	Route of administration	Dose mg/kg (except as indicated)	Hours between doses
Penicillin G, benzathine	im	40,000 U/kg	72–120

Notes: Suboptimal drug concentrations possible.

Penicillin V	po	10	8

Notes: Substitute for penicillin G when oral administration preferred.

Cloxacillin	po,iv,im	30	8

Notes: Active against penicillinase-producing staphylococci, unlike penicillins G or V.

Penicillins, wider spectrum

Ampicillin	po	10–20	8–12
	iv,im,sc	5–10	8
Amoxycillin	po	10–20	12–24
	iv,im,sc	5–10	12–24
Amoxycillin-clavulanate	po	12.5–25 (combined)	12–24

Notes: Bactericidal, excreted in urine. Ampicillin is less active than penicillin G against anaerobic Gram-positive facultative species, but more active against Gram-negative facultative bacilli. Amoxycillin has similar spectrum but better oral bioavailability. Combining amoxycillin with clavulanate widens the antibacterial spectrum by protecting amoxycillin from some β-lactamases.

Fluoroquinolones

Ciprofloxacin	po	5–15	12
Enrofloxacin	po	2.5–10	12
Norfloxacin	po	5–20	12

Notes: Bactericidal, active against Gram-negative aerobic and facultative bacteria, some staphylococci and some corynebacteria. Little activity against streptococci and anaerobic pathogens. Well distributed to tissues and body fluids. Partially metabolized by liver and excreted in bile or urine partly as active drug or metabolites. Possible side-effects: vomiting, diarrhoea, nephrotoxicity, and cartilage defects in prepubertal patients. Use lower dose for urinary infections, higher for soft tissue infections, osteomyelitis.

Sulphonamides and potentiators

Sulfadiazine	po	50–100	12
Sulfadiazine–trimethoprim	po,iv,im,sc	30 (combined)	24

Table 3.4 Continued

Drugs	Route of administration	Dose mg/kg (except as indicated)	Hours between doses
Sulfadimethoxine	po,iv,im,sc	25	12–24
Pyrimethamine	po	0.5–1	24

Notes: Sulphonamides (bacteriostatic, broad spectrum) now rarely used alone. Trimethoprim enhances antibacterial activity. Occasional adverse effects reported in cats: salivation, vomiting, ataxia, seizures, depression, disorientation. Also (in dogs): dry eye, skin reactions, polyarthritis. Potential folate deficiency. Pyrimethamine improves antiprotozoal efficacy of sulphonamides but is unpalatable to cats: the combination may cause depression, anorexia, and reversible bone marrow suppression.

Tetracyclines			
Doxycycline	po,iv	3–5	12
Minocycline	po	5–15	12
Oxytetracycline	po	20	8
	iv,im	10	12
Tetracycline	po	25	8

Notes: Bacteriostatic. Active against many Gram-positive and Gram-negative bacteria, also rickettsia, mycoplasma, chlamydia, protozoa. Oral administration preferred, painful im. Excreted mainly as active drug in urine, some in bile. Doxycycline eliminated mainly in faeces. Doxycycline and minocycline penetrate tissues best. Side-effects: gastrointestinal upsets, anorexia, pyrexia, tooth discoloration, (avoid in last third of pregnancy, first month of life).

Miscellaneous antimicrobials			
Chloramphenicol	po	12–20	12
	iv,im,sc	20–30	12

Notes: Bacteriostatic, broad spectrum, including anaerobes, mycoplasma, rickettsia, chlamydia. Distributed widely *in vivo*. Metabolized by liver, excreted in urine (25% in active form). Indicated oral dose safe for 3 weeks, higher dose (20 mg/kg, repeat 8 h) possible up to 1 week. Side-effects: depression, inappetence, vomiting, diarrhoea, reversible marrow suppression.

Dapsone	po	1	8–12

Notes: Required dose rate uncertain. May cause haemolysis, neurotoxicity.

Furazolidone	po	4	12

Table 3.4 Continued

Drugs	Route of administration	Dose mg/kg (except as indicated)	Hours between doses
Metronidazole	po	10–25	12–24
Notes: For giardiosis.			
		10–15	8
Notes: For anaerobic bacterial infections.			
Quinacrine	po	5–10	12–24
Rifampicin	po	10–20	12
Notes: Required dose rate uncertain.			

iv, Intravenous; im, intramuscular; po, by mouth; sc, subcutaneous.

OUTCOME

The most satisfying response to antimicrobial therapy occurs when the correct drug is used to treat an uncomplicated microbial infection in a patient that is otherwise well. In contrast, the outcome is likely to be disappointing if the wrong drug is chosen, if microbes are not responsible (or viruses are), or if complicating factors have not been addressed. Additional specific or supportive measures, such as nursing, fluid therapy and surgery, might also be needed.

The treatment regimen should be re-evaluated if there is no response to conventional dosage within a 48-h period; selection of a different drug might then be warranted, but increased dosage with the initial drug could be considered if poor tissue penetration is suspected.

If the response to appropriate therapy is poor, or repeated relapses occur, the possibility of underlying immunodeficiency caused by feline leukaemia virus or feline immunodeficiency virus should be investigated.

ACKNOWLEDGEMENTS

The assistance of Dr D. N. Love in preparing the table on anti-microbial drug selection is gratefully acknowledged. Data in this article were compiled from the various references listed.

REFERENCES AND FURTHER READING

Aucoin, D. (1993) *Target*. Port Huron, North American Compendiums.

Boothe, D. M. (1989) The practical aspects of treating bacterial infection in cats. *Veterinary Medicine* **84**, 885–904.

Boothe, D. M. (1990) Drug therapy in cats (4 parts). *Journal of the American Veterinary Medical Association* **196**, 1297–1305, 1502–1511, 1659–1669, 1845–1850.

Brancker, W. M. (1962) The sedation of cats. *Advances in Small Animal Practice (Proceedings of BSAVA)* **4**, 9.

Greene, C. E. (ed.) (1990) *Infectious Diseases of the Dog and Cat*. Philadelphia, W. B. Saunders.

Holzworth, J. & Stein, B. S. (1987) The sick cat. In: *Diseases of the Cat, Medicine and Surgery* (ed. J. Holzworth), pp. 9–13. Philadelphia, W. B. Saunders.

Lorenz, M. D., Cornelius, L. M. & Ferguson, D. C. (eds) (1993) *Small Animal Medical Therapeutics*. Philadelphia, J. B. Lippincott.

Prescott, J. F. & Baggot, J. D. (1988) *Antimicrobial Therapy in Veterinary Medicine*. Boston, Blackwell.

CHAPTER 4

Differential Diagnosis of Uveitis

CHERIDA HOPPER AND SHEILA CRISPIN

INTRODUCTION

Uveitis refers to inflammation of the uveal tract. This may involve:

(1) The anterior uvea, i.e. the iris (iritis) or iris and anterior part (pars plicata) or the ciliary body (iridocyclitis)
(2) The pars plana of the ciliary body (pars planitis or intermediate uveitis)
(3) The posterior uvea, i.e. the choroid (choroiditis or chorioretinitis)
(4) The whole of the uveal tract (panuveitis).

Uveitis is an important and relatively common clinical presentation in the cat. The aetiology involves both infectious and non-infectious causes and, in contrast to uveitis in the dog, feline uveitis is often caused by infectious agents. Acute uveitis is often less painful in cats than dogs and therefore in many cases the condition may already be becoming chronic before the cat is presented to the veterinary surgeon. Consequently, helpful clues from both the history and early ophthalmic examination may be unavailable. Nevertheless, it is necessary to try and establish the cause of every case of uveitis, not only to enable specific therapy to be used, if appropriate, but also to make an accurate prognosis for the cat concerned and to provide the correct advice regarding management of other cats in the household.

CLINICAL PRESENTATION OF UVEITIS

It is important to know the appearance of the healthy feline eye (Fig. 4.1) and to remember that in all cases both eyes should be examined carefully and the findings compared.

The clinical presentation varies according to the extent of uveal tract involvement and whether the condition is acute or chronic. A summary of the clinical findings is given in Tables 4.1 and 4.2.

Acute anterior uveitis is associated with varying degrees of pain. When pain is marked there is usually accompanying blepharospasm, excessive lacrimation and photophobia, although these clinical signs are never as intense as those observed in some canine cases. The eye is reddened, mainly because of active hyperaemia of the circumferentially arranged episcleral vessels. Corneal oedema is usually present and occasionally keratic precipitates may be observed adhering to the posterior surface of the cornea; marked aqueous flare is

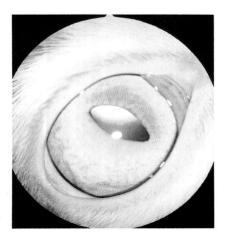

Fig. 4.1
Appearance of a normal eye in a healthy cat.

Table 4.1 Clinical signs of anterior uveitis in the cat.

Feature	Acute	Chronic
Pain	+ to + + +	− to +
Redness	+ + to + + +	− to +
Cornea	May be oedematous	Possibly local opacities
Aqueous flare	+ + to + + +	− to +
Keratic precipitates/mutton fat deposits	Occasionally	Frequently
Anterior chamber	Normal to aqueous flare	KPs/hypopyon/ hyphaema
Iris	Congested; difficult to observe fine detail	Darkened, rubeosis iridis, iris nodules
Pupil shape	Normal to miotic	Normal to eccentric
Pupil response	Poor response to light	Normal/partial/fixed
Intraocular pressure	Low to normal	Usually normal
Lens	Normal except opacities at sites of posterior synechiae	Normal to cataractous; posterior synechiae; pigment deposition
Vision	Normal/impaired/blind	Usually normal

−, Absent; +, mild; + +, moderate; + + +, severe; KP, keratic precipitate.

characteristic of the acute situation. Fibrin clots may form within the anterior chamber and haemorrhage may also occur in some cases. The iris is typically thickened and the fine detail of its surface architecture is lost; inflammation of the iris vessels can be observed directly with magnification. Synechiae may form rapidly and, if the globe is intact, posterior synechiae are usual. If rupture of the globe has occurred, however, the sudden loss of intraocular pressure and the release of aqueous humour may bring the iris and cornea into apposition so that anterior synechiae form. Occasionally, the iris may prolapse through the full-thickness perforation and, rarely, there may be expulsive loss of the intraocular contents. Other features which may be present include reduced intraocular pressure, miosis and a reduced or absent pupillary light response. Vision may be impaired or the cat may be blind.

Table 4.2 Clinical signs of posterior uveitis in the cat.

Feature	Acute	Chronic
Vitreous	May be cloudy because of cellular infiltration/ haemorrhage	Usually clear, but possibly cellular infiltration/ haemorrhage
Retina	Initially not involved unless intense choroidal inflammation and subretinal exudation	Secondary involvement – inflammation/haemorrhage/ detachment
Choroid	Focal and diffuse choroiditis	Changes in colour, texture and pigmentation
Optic nerve	Normal to optic neuritis; may be peripapillary haemorrhage	Normal to optic atrophy
Vision	Normal/impaired/blind	Normal/impaired/blind

Acute intermediate uveitis is rarely diagnosed as it produces little, if any, ocular pain and, initially, inflammatory cells are located near the pars plana which is not very accessible to ophthalmoscopic examination.

Acute posterior uveitis may occur with or without obvious involvement of the anterior uvea. Characteristic features include chorioretinitis lesions, which are often focal and rather subtle in acute cases, with accompanying local oedema and haemorrhage. Retinal detachment is a common complication and optic neuritis occurs in some cases. Vision may be reduced or absent.

Chronic anterior uveitis is associated with the formation of keratic precipitates and, sometimes, the larger "mutton fat" deposits. Such precipitates and deposits are most obvious on the ventral aspect of the posterior cornea. A variety of anterior chamber deposits may be encountered, with hyphaema and hypopyon being the most common. Iris neovascularization (rubeosis iridis) is a readily observed feature of chronic iritis in cats, as are iris nodules, which are a consequence of lymphoid hyperplasia. The colour of the iris is darker in established cases. Irregularity of pupil shape with an imperfect response to bright light is a common feature of chronic uveitis and usually indicates established posterior synechiae. Pigment deposits on the anterior lens capsule (iris rests) are a legacy of previous iris inflammation. Ectropion uveae and, rarely, uveal cysts may be present and cataracts may form secondary to the uveitis. Occasionally, lens luxation is a sequel to chronic anterior uveitis but, in the cat, unlike the dog, it is very unusual for this to lead to glaucoma.

Chronic intermediate uveitis is characterized by "snowball opacities" near the pars plana, on the posterior lens capsule and within the anterior vitreous.

Chronic posterior uveitis can present as a non-specific diffuse or focal chorioretinopathy. Chronic changes include aberrant fundic pigmentation and a fundus of granular appearance. Both recent and older retinal haemorrhage may be observed and extensive intraocular haemorrhage is sometimes seen. Partial or complete retinal detachment and optic atrophy may also be present.

CONDITIONS RESEMBLING UVEITIS

A number of conditions, including conjunctivitis, keratitis, persistent pupillary membranes, glaucoma and neoplasia, may superficially resemble uveitis and must be differentiated from it (Table 4.3).

CAUSES OF FELINE UVEITIS

The causes of feline uveitis are listed in Table 4.4 and described in detail in the text.

NON-INFECTIOUS CAUSES

Blunt trauma

Any blow to the head may result in the release of intraocular inflammatory mediators, such as prostaglandins, and hence to the development of uveitis. In cats the most common cause of such an injury is a road traffic accident and careful questioning

Table 4.3 Conditions resembling uveitis.

Condition	Ocular appearance
Conjunctivitis	Ocular redness – acute cases show conjunctival hyperaemia and usually chemosis and ocular discharge (Fig. 4.2). Intraocular appearance should be normal
Keratitis	Corneal opacity because of generalized or localized corneal inflammation (must be distinguished from corneal oedema, aqueous flare and keratic precipitates associated with uveitis). NB Superficial keratitis (Fig. 4.3) is not usually associated with uveitis, but deep keratitis (Fig. 4.4) often causes mild anterior uveitis
Congenital conditions	e.g. Persistent pupillary membrane (Fig. 4.5) may resemble anterior synechiae, and other abnormalities of mesodermal differentiation may be confused with anterior uveitis
Glaucoma	Typically, a fixed, dilated pupil with elevated intraocular pressure ± globe enlargement. Pain and reddening of the eye may not be apparent in cats (Fig. 4.6). Glaucoma following uveitis (Fig. 4.7) is less common in cats than dogs – occurs, e.g., when neoplastic or inflammatory cells block filtration angle
Neoplasia	Solid tumours or diffuse infiltrate can mimic uveitis, or be a cause of uveitis (see later)
Primary tumours	e.g. Uveal melanoma (Fig. 4.8), adenoma, adenocarcinoma, leiomyoma (Fig. 4.9) – usually form unilateral discrete masses, but can be diffuse
Secondary tumours	The most common is multicentric lymphoma (Fig. 4.10) (often FeLV associated). Others include carcinoma, sarcoma, reticulosis and plasma cell myeloma. All may form well-defined uveal masses or may be diffuse, closely resembling uveitis
Orbital and optic nerve tumours	e.g. Meningioma, glioma, astrocytoma, can extend into the eye producing a range of intraocular and extraocular effects

of the owner and thorough examination of the cat are necessary before trauma can be discounted.

One or both eyes may be affected, depending on the location of the injury, but it is more commonly a unilateral presentation. The whole of the uveal tract is usually involved, most often

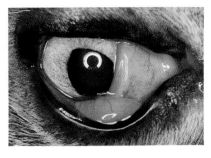

Fig. 4.2
A domestic shorthaired (DSH) cat with acute conjunctivitis, characterized by ocular discharge, conjunctival hyperaemia and chemosis.

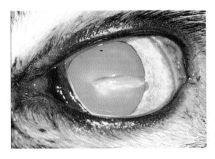

Fig. 4.3
Acute superficial corneal ulcer, resulting from a cat scratch, stained with fluorescein.

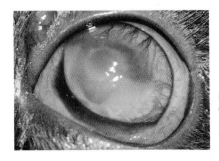

Fig. 4.4
Chronic, deep corneal ulcer in a Persian cat which had inadvertently been treated with corticosteroid. The brown area represents corneal necrosis. This cat also had low-grade anterior uveitis.

in an acute inflammatory response, and typical signs include aqueous flare, hyphaema, miosis, iris thickening, posterior synechiae formation, retinal oedema and/or, haemorrhage, retinal detachment and reduced intraocular pressure. Blindness may occur either as a consequence of the retinal lesions or because of central damage. There is usually a degree of pain with accompanying photophobia and blepharospasm. Blunt trauma may lead to cataract formation in some cases (Fig. 4.11). Occasionally, there may be a considerable delay between the traumatic incident and the onset of signs of uveitis.

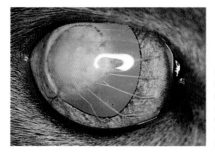

Fig. 4.5
Persistent pupillary membrane in a young DSH cat. The mesodermal remnants pass from the iris collarette to the posterior cornea. Corneal opacification is a consequence of interference with endothelial metabolism. Some of the vascular channels remain patent so there is also corneal vascularization.

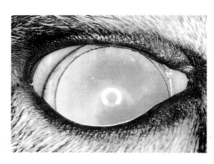

Fig. 4.6
Primary glaucoma in a DSH cat. The pupil is widely dilated but there is no episcleral or conjunctival congestion and the eye is not painful.

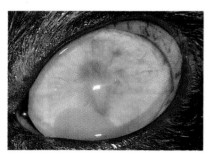

Fig. 4.7
Chronic uveitis with secondary glaucoma. The pupil is fixed and eccentric, with extensive posterior synechiae; there is cataract formation in the lens and also a white coloured deposit in the anterior chamber.

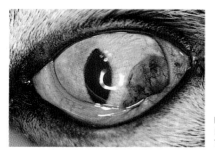

Fig. 4.8
Iris melanoma affecting the right eye of a DSH cat. There is an intense perilimbal vascular response.

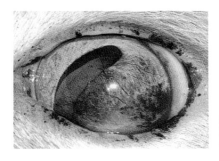

Fig. 4.9
DSH cat with leiomyoma arising from the ciliary body and infiltrating the iris.

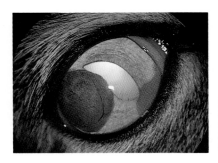

Fig. 4.10
Multicentric lymphoma in a DSH cat. There is a solid mass in the upper outer aspect of the anterior chamber and liquid neoplastic infiltrate in the ventral aspect of the anterior chamber.

Table 4.4 Important causes of feline uveitis.

Non-infectious	Viral parasitic	Mycotic
Blunt trauma	FeLV toxoplasmosis	Cryptococcosis
Penetrating trauma	FIP	Histoplasmosis
Deep keratitis	FIV	Blastomycosis
Neoplasia		

Penetrating trauma

Penetrating and perforating ocular injuries arise most commonly from cat fights, and occasionally from foreign bodies and gun-shot wounds. The lesions are almost always unilateral. As with blunt trauma, an acute uveitis results from the release of inflammatory mediators. In addition, the release of protein from cells damaged by direct trauma, e.g. lens protein, may induce an autoimmune uveitis. The clinical appearance is very variable

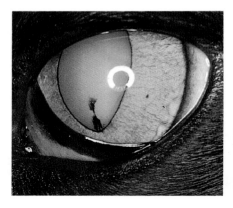

Fig. 4.11
Cataract formation 8 months after blunt ocular trauma. The uveitis which occurred at the time of trauma has resolved leaving iris rests which indicate the site of previous adhesions between iris and lens.

and relates to the extent and nature of the ocular damage. Intra-corneal foreign bodies often cause minimal inflammation while perforation of the globe usually results in a reddened, uncomfortable eye with an intense uveitis (Fig. 4.12). If a perfor-ating injury is not recognized and treated, possible sequelae include intraocular infection, iris prolapse and glaucoma. Even with appropriate action it is not unusual to see some legacy of previous inflammation, e.g. posterior synechiae, irregularity of pupil shape and alteration in the colour of the iris (Fig. 4.13). Direct trauma to the lens may lead to cataract formation.

Neoplasia

All presentations of uveitis, ranging from acute to chronic, anterior to posterior, may occur in association with ocular tumours. However, as a general' rule, neoplasia should be sus-pected in cases where there is marked iris thickening, alteration

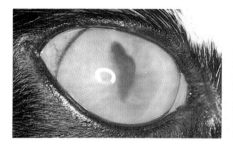

Fig. 4.12
DSH cat approximately 1 week after a cat fight, during which there was full-thickness penetration of the cornea. The site of penetration can be seen immediately beneath the markedly eccentric and constricted pupil. The details of the iris are unclear because of an anterior chamber exudate and iris oedema.

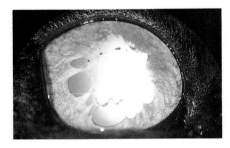

Fig. 4.13
Highly irregular pupil shape, darkening of the iris, and posterior synechiae as a result of previous trauma in a DSH cat. Compare the arrangement of the synechiae in this case with the persistent pupillary membrane of Fig. 4.5.

in iris pigmentation, an anterior chamber infiltrate, or intra-ocular haemorrhage.

Corneal injury

A transient and usually mild uveitis, known as reflex uveitis, may immediately follow corneal injury. In the patient shown in Fig. 4.14, reflex uveitis is a consequence of a corneal foreign body. A more marked and prolonged anterior uveitis may be induced by the presence of deep keratitis (for example, severe corneal ulceration).

Idiopathic uveitis

Failure to identify a specific cause of uveitis, despite extensive laboratory investigations, is not uncommon. Such cases are

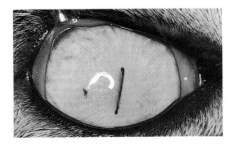

Fig. 4.14
DSH cat which has a thorn (seen at lateral tip of camera flash) embedded in the cornea. Reflex iritis followed the injury.

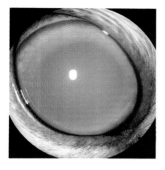

Fig. 4.15
Unilateral panuveitis of acute onset in a 16-month-old chinchilla cat
with neurological signs. No cause was established for either problem
and both resolved within a month.

termed idiopathic (Figs 4.15 and 4.16). Some of the cases of
unknown aetiology may be related to underlying systemic
infection which has defied detection (see later). It is possible
that other cases could be associated with infectious agents that
have yet to be characterized. Another potential cause is
immune-mediated uveitis, which has been induced experimen-
tally in response to a variety of circulating antigens.

INFECTIOUS CAUSES

Viral causes of uveitis

Feline infectious peritonitis virus (FIPV)

FIP is one of the most common diagnoses associated with
uveitis in cats. Both wet and dry forms of the disease may be

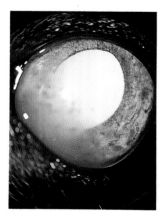

Fig. 4.16
A 13-year-old DSH cat with chronic bilateral uveitis of unknown
cause.

accompanied by ophthalmic signs, although uveitis is much more commonly found in dry FIP. It may be the principal lesion in many cases of dry FIP. Some clues may be gained from the history because FIP is found more frequently in younger cats than older cats and is most common in pedigree cats kept in multicat households. Non-ophthalmic signs are very variable but usually include non-specific signs of illness such as lethargy, pyrexia, inappetence and weight loss. In a typical wet (or effusive) case, ascites and/or, thoracic effusion should become apparent. In dry FIP, progressive neurological signs relating to brain and spinal cord lesions commonly occur. The ocular lesions of FIP almost invariably involve the anterior uveal tract (Fig. 4.17) and may also affect the posterior uvea. Both eyes are often involved, although usually the lesions are not bilaterally symmetrical. The pathogenesis is associated with perivascular pyogranulomatous inflammation and subsequent breakdown of the blood–aqueous barrier. Inflammatory cells and plasma proteins, such as fibrin, leak into the aqueous or vitreous humour, giving rise to hypopyon, keratic precipitates and aqueous flare or vitreous opacity. Rubeosis iridis is often apparent and there may be microhaemorrhages from the inflamed vessels, and sometimes frank hyphaema (Fig. 4.18). If it is possible to examine the fundus, focal or diffuse areas of chorioretinitis, with accompanying retinal oedema and/or, haemorrhage, may be present. Retinal detachment can occur in some cases.

Feline leukaemia virus (FeLV)

Uveitis is the most common ocular manifestation of FeLV infection and almost any presentation may occur. Cats of all ages

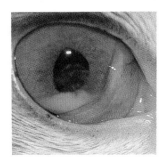

Fig. 4.17
Chronic bilateral uveitis in a 6-month-old DSH cat. There is fibrin in the dorsal pupillary aperture and a cellular exudate in the ventral anterior chamber. FIP was suspected and confirmed post-mortem.

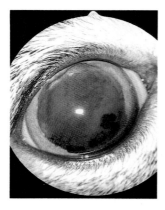

Fig. 4.18
Frank hyphaema obscuring signs of chronic uveitis in a DSH cat with FIP (confirmed post-mortem).

may be affected although FeLV infection is much more common in young cats and is rare in cats over 10 years of age. Discrete FeLV-induced lymphomatous tumours of the anterior uvea are usually accompanied by a degree of localized uveitis (see section on neoplasia). In such cases, uveitis can be bilateral although the changes in the non-tumorous eye may be very subtle. Ocular lymphoma is most frequently accompanied by involvement of other organs and thorough clinical examination and radiography are necessary to establish the extent of the lesions. Chronic uveitis can occur as a result of generalized uveal infiltration by neoplastic cells. Immune-mediated inflammation in response to immune complex deposition may also be involved in the pathogenesis. Aqueous flare, keratic precipitates, hypopyon, rubeosis iridis, hyphaema, anterior and posterior synechiae, and thickening and pigmentary changes of the iris are the most frequently observed signs (Figs 4.19 and 4.20). Secondary glaucoma may arise because neoplastic and inflammatory cells obstruct the drainage angle. Posterior segment changes occur less frequently and, in addition, may be difficult or impossible to observe because of anterior uveal lesions. Vitreous opacities sometimes develop and a variety of fundic lesions including tumour infiltration, pigment proliferation, retinal degeneration, retinal haemorrhage, partial or complete retinal detachment and optic neuritis, may be present.

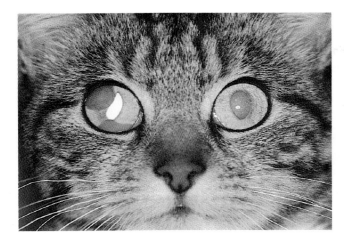

Fig. 4.19
Non-symmetrical, bilateral uveitis in a cat with FeLV infection. The right eye is shown in detail in Fig. 4.9. The left eye shows marked aqueous flare and some keratic precipitates are also present.

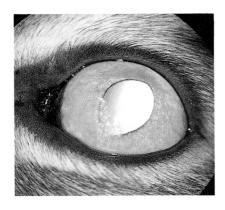

Fig. 4.20
Low grade iritis in a young cat with FeLV infection. There are numerous keratic precipitates which are particularly obvious adhering to the back of the cornea in the ventromedial quadrant.

Feline immunodeficiency virus (FIV)

A significant proportion of cats with uveitis are infected with FIV, usually in the absence of infection with any other agent commonly associated with uveitis. The pathogenesis of uveal lesions is unclear but may be related to immune-mediated mechanisms, e.g. through the deposition of immune complexes, or to the localization of FIV in uveal lymphoid tissue. Cats in the later stages of FIV infection may develop uveitis as a result of secondary infection with a variety of organisms, including FIPV and *Toxoplasma gondii*, although at present this is not frequently observed. FIV occurs most often in adult, free-roaming,

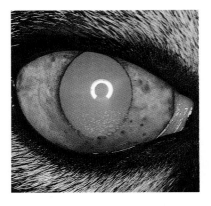

Fig. 4.21
Chronic unilateral uveitis in a six-year-old DSH cat infected with FIV. Keratic precipitates are evident in the ventromedial quadrant.

non-pedigree cats and is more common in males than females. Clinical problems associated with FIV infection rarely occur in isolation and other signs, together with haematological changes such as lymphopenia and anaemia, may be evident. Cats may present with acute uveitis but chronic or recurrent uveitis is more usual and some cases present with pars planitis. Clinically, there is no distinction between lesions associated with FIV and those relating to FIPV or FeLV infection. Corneal oedema, keratic precipitates, aqueous flare, hypopyon, irregularity of pupil size, iris thickening, rubeosis iridis, synechiae formation and hyphaema may all be present (Figs 4.21 and 4.22). Intermediate and posterior lesions include planitis (Fig. 4.23), focal chorioretinitis, retinal haemorrhage and retinal detachment (Fig. 4.24).

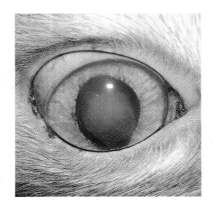

Fig. 4.22
Chronic bilateral uveitis in a DSH cat with FIV infection. Protruding through the pupil is a large fibrin clot; ventrally there is blood incorporated into the clot.

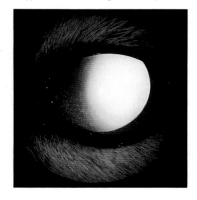

Fig. 4.23
DSH cat with pars planitis. The opacities are adherent to the posterior lens capsule.

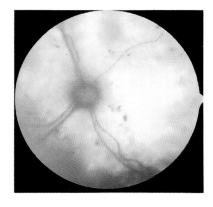

Fig. 4.24
Fundus of a 15-year-old British blue with FIV infection of at least 4 years' duration. Hypertensive changes are present in both eyes. In this eye there are multiple focal retinal haemorrhages and abnormal retinal vessels (note especially the focal narrowing with disruption of the blood column which is present in the arteriole between 1 and 2 o'clock. The other eye had a serious exudative retinal detachment which resulted in acute vision loss. The hypertension was probably unrelated to the FIV infection.

Parasitic causes of uveitis

Toxoplasmosis

Toxoplasma gondii is an intracellular coccidian parasite found throughout the world. The domestic cat and other felidae are the only definitive hosts, whereas any mammal may act as the intermediate host. The life cycle is very complex and is given in detail elsewhere (Dubey, 1986). Clinical signs of toxoplasma infection are uncommon in the cat, both in the acute primary phase of infection and in chronic secondary toxoplasmosis which follows the recrudescence of encysted organisms. When disease does occur, a wide range of clinical signs may develop, including pyrexia, weight loss, diarrhoea, vomiting, uveitis, neurological and respiratory signs. Any form of immunosuppression is likely to predispose to the development of disease. Ocular lesions are rare in acute disease but frequently occur in chronic toxoplasmosis. Posterior uveitis, anterior uveitis and panuveitis have all been documented; lesions may be unilateral or bilateral. Early reports established that the principal lesion was posterior uveitis, while involvement of the anterior uvea was thought to occur mainly in the later stages of the disease, and only in a proportion of cases. However, in contrast, a recent report of clinical toxoplasmosis (Lappin *et al.*, 1989) found that anterior uveal lesions were more frequent than those in the posterior uvea. Anterior uveitis is chronic in nature and can result from granulomatous infiltration or a hypersensitivity reaction of the iris. The appearance is clinically indistinguishable from other forms of infectious uveitis. Fundus changes consist of multifocal, or occasionally generalized, chorioretinitis lesions which may be granulomatous or non-granulomatous. There may be associated exudative (bullous) retinal detachments (Fig. 4.25). Old, inactive focal chorioretinopathies may coexist with active lesions.

Mycotic uveitis

Three fungal infections are associated with uveitis in cats – cryptococcosis, histoplasmosis and blastomycosis. However, reports of these infections are rare and tend to be limited to countries where mycoses are endemic. They are very unlikely to occur in the UK unless the cat has been imported from such

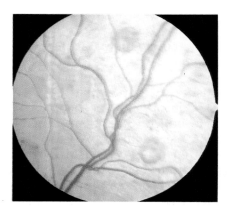

Fig. 4.25
Fundus of a cat with toxoplasmosis showing focal retinitis lesions ventrally and circular areas of bullous retinal detachment more dorsally.

a country. Nevertheless, when presented with a case of uveitis, it is always worth asking the owner if the cat has been abroad at any time in the past. Salient details of the infections are given in Table 4.5. All three species of fungi have yeast forms capable of growth in animal tissues. In general, ocular lesions occur only when the infection becomes systemic. The principal lesion involves the fundus (Fig. 4.26), and the anterior uvea may not be involved at all, or only in the later stages of the disease. The lesions are almost always bilateral, but are rarely symmetrical. It is not possible to distinguish between these three infections by ocular examination.

Miscellaneous forms of infectious uveitis

Bacterial causes of uveitis are virtually non-existent in the cat. Isolated cases of uveitis associated with tuberculosis are the exception. Other very rare causes include aberrant nematodes, candidiasis and infection with *Coccidioides immitis*, a soil fungus found in the south-western United States and parts of Central and South America.

DIAGNOSTIC APPROACH

Obtaining a diagnosis for uveitis in the cat can be a considerable challenge because a great range of presentations may occur, particularly in association with the infectious causes, and none is specifically associated with any single aetiology.

When investigating a case it is vital first to take a detailed history and then to perform a thorough clinical and ophthalmic examination. Unless the uveitis is obviously traumatic in origin, all cases should be tested for FeLV, FIV and coronavirus. Should the results prove unhelpful, toxoplasma serology should also be carried out and, on the few occasions where the history is appropriate, tests for the mycotic infections may be useful (see below for limitations of diagnosis).

It is advisable, if financial considerations permit, to assess haematology and blood biochemistry while taking blood samples for serodiagnosis. If FIP is suspected, serum protein analysis and serum protein electrophoresis are specifically

Table 4.5 Details of the commonest mycotic infections in cats.

Organism	Endemic areas	Pre-dispositions	Location of lesions	Non-ocular signs	Ocular signs
Cryptococcus neoformans (most common)	Mainly USA	None	Respiratory tract, followed by skin, eye and central nervous system	Relate to site of lesions	Posterior – dark, raised focal granulomata, or generalized chorioretinitis with haemorrhage and retinal detachment. Anterior – only in few cases
Histoplasma capsulatum	Temperate and tropical river valleys	Young cats	Respiratory tract mainly	Relate to site of lesions	Posterior – focal granulomatous chorioretinitis. Anterior – very rare
Blastomyces dermatitidis (rare)	North America (also Africa and South America)	None	Respiratory tract mainly	Relate to site of lesions. Terminal weight loss, pyrexia and depression	Posterior – grey-white choroidal granulomata. Anterior – chronic granulomatous uveitis

NB These organisms do not occur in the UK and will only be found in animals which have lived in endemic areas.

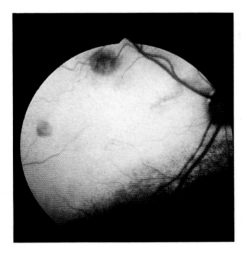

Fig. 4.26
Two chronic, focal granulomatous lesions in the fundus of a Siamese cat which presented with a large, reddened, fleshy lesion of one upper eyelid. Because the cat had lived in Venezuela and New York before being imported into the UK, a mycotic infection was suspected and *Cryptococcus neoformans* was cultured from a biopsy of the eyelid lesion.

recommended, and should be carried out if at all possible. Other investigative techniques, such as radiography, ultrasonography and abdominal paracentesis, may be informative in appropriate cases. A guide to the investigation of uveitis is given in Table 4.6.

Ultimately, if the uveitis and/or, other associated problems become very severe, histopathology, either of an enucleated eye, or of eye and other body tissues taken post mortem, may provide a definitive diagnosis.

LIMITATIONS OF SERODIAGNOSIS

Unfortunately the results of serodiagnosis, with the possible exception of FeLV testing, are not always clear cut and the problems are outlined briefly below.

Table 4.6 Diagnostic aids in the investigation of feline uveitis.

Investigation	Relevance
History	Age, breed, sex predispositions for infections? Additional clinical signs? Suggestion of trauma? Imported from abroad?
Clinical examination	
Ophthalmic	Uveitis – acute/chronic; anterior/intermediate/ posterior; unilateral/bilateral? Associated ophthalmic problems?
General	Additional clinical problems? – signs of trauma – signs of systemic infection – signs of neoplasia
Serodiagnosis*	
FeLV/FIV/ coronavirus	Diagnose/rule out FeLV; diagnose FIV; gain indication of FIP
Toxoplasma	Gain indication of toxoplasma infection
(Mycotic species)	(Indication of mycotic infection, if appropriate)
Haematology	Indication of viral infection Indication of chronic inflammation/systemic infection
Serum biochemistry	
Routine	Indication of additional clinical problems
Protein electrophoresis	Hypergammaglobulinaemia associated with FIP, lymphocytic cholangitis, FIV and toxoplasmosis Raised alpha-2-globulins associated with FIV and FIP
Abdominal paracentesis	If appropriate. Protein rich, straw-coloured fluid which clots is typical of wet FIP
Radiography	If suspected ocular tumour present. Chest radiographs to look for metastasis
Ultrasonography	If intraocular examination difficult. To identify intraocular neoplasia/intraocular haemorrhage/retinal detachment

* See text for limitations of serodiagnosis.

FIV

Routine testing involves the detection of antibody to FIV and a positive result is conclusive. However, a significant proportion of infected cats do not have detectable antibody and therefore a negative antibody result does not rule out FIV infection.

FIP

Interpretations of "FIP" serology is notoriously difficult for several reasons. First, cats may be infected by a number of coronaviruses other than feline infectious peritonitis virus (FIPV) — principally feline enteric coronavirus (FECV), but also canine coronavirus and transmissible gastroenteritis virus (TGEV) of pigs. Antibodies to all these viruses cross-react and it is impossible to determine whether a cat has antibody to FIPV or to one of the other coronaviruses. Second, although cats with confirmed FIP often have high coronavirus titres, low and even zero titres may occur. In addition, many healthy cats have high titres. Third, titres may vary according to which diagnostic technique (and laboratory) is used. Consequently, a high coronavirus titre in a case of uveitis, together with an appropriate history, may be strongly suggestive of FIP, but an intermediate, low or negative titre does not rule out infection. Ultimately, FIP can be confirmed only by histological examination of biopsy or post mortem tissues.

Toxoplasmosis

Standard testing for toxoplasma involves the detection of IgG antibodies to the organism. This test is unhelpful in demonstrating active toxoplasmosis because IgG levels take at least a month to rise following initial infection, and remain high for up to a year. The IgG titres also remain high following recrudescence of toxoplasma. Misunderstanding of these facts can lead to the incorrect diagnosis of toxoplasmosis in cases of uveitis. Paired serum sampling may be more helpful and a fourfold rise over 2–3 weeks is suggestive of active infection. IgM antibody levels provide a more accurate indication of active infection, as they rise within 2 weeks of infection and become negative after

16 weeks. It is important to use the same laboratory for the analysis of paired samples because titres can vary markedly according to the method of antibody detection.

Mycotic infections

Serological diagnosis of mycotic infections is not readily available in the UK. If non-ocular manifestations of mycotic infection are present then the most reliable method of diagnosis is microscopic identification and/or, fungal culture of a biopsy, smear or aspirate of the lesion.

ACKNOWLEDGEMENTS

The authors would like to thank J. Conibear and M. Parsons for their photographic assistance and J. P. Oleshko for permission to use Fig. 4.8. Cherida Hopper was supported by the Wellcome Trust.

REFERENCES AND FURTHER READING

Barlough, J. E. & Stoddart, C. A. (1988) Cats and coronaviruses. *Journal of the American Veterinary Medical Association* **193**, 796–800.

Blouin, P. (1984) Uveitis in the dog and cat: causes, diagnosis and treatment. *Canadian Veterinary Journal* **25**, 315–323.

Chavkin, M. J., Lappin, M. R., Powell, C. C., Roberts, S. M., Parshall, C. J. & Reif, J. S. (1992) Seroepidemiologic and clinical observations of 93 cases of uveitis in cats. *Progress in Veterinary and Comparative Ophthalmology* **2**, 29–36.

Crispin, S. M. (1988) Uveitis in the dog and cat. *Journal of Small Animal Practice* **29**, 429–447.

Dubey, J. P. (1986) Toxoplasmosis in cats. *Feline Practice* **16**, 12–16, 18–45.

English, R. V., Davidson, M. G., Nasisse, M. P., Jamieson, V. E. & Lappin, M. R. (1990) Intraocular disease associated with feline immunodeficiency virus infection in cats. *Journal of the American Veterinary Medical Association* **196**, 1116–1119.

Lappin, M. R., Greene, C. E., Winston, S., Toll, S. L. & Epstein, M. E. (1989) Clinical feline toxoplasmosis. *Journal of Veterinary Internal Medicine* **3**, 139–143.

Legendre, A. M. (1989) Systemic mycotic infections. In: *The Cat: Diseases and Clinical Management* (ed. Sherding, R. G.), pp. 427–437. New York, Churchill Livingstone.

Pfeiffer, R. L. & Wilcock, B. P. (1991) Histopathologic study of uveitis in cats: 139 cases (1978–1988). *Journal of the American Veterinary Medical Association* **198**, 135–138.

Williams, L. W., Gelatti, K. N. & Ewin, R. M. (1981) Ophthalmic neoplasms in the cat. *Journal of the American Animal Hospital Association* **17**, 999–1008.

CHAPTER 5

Feline Neurology Part 1: Intracranial Disorders

ANDREW HOPKINS

INTRODUCTION

An understanding of the principles of lesion localization is essential for the correct diagnosis and management of all neurological problems. This topic is covered thoroughly by De Lahunta (1983) and Oliver *et al.* (1987) and will not be discussed here. It is the author's intention to provide the reader with an easily recalled set of differential diagnoses following lesion localization which will act as a guide to the investigation of feline neurological diseases.

The neurological signs assist in broadly localizing lesions to the brain, spinal cord and neuromuscular system. The brain and spinal cord constitute the central nervous system (CNS). The term neuromuscular system encompasses the peripheral nerve, neuromuscular junction and muscle cell, disorders of which may be referred to as neuropathy, junctionopathy and myopathy, respectively. Some disease processes give rise to multifocal lesions and the recognition of multifocal signs often aids in narrowing the diagnostic possibilities.

Neurological diseases involve five major pathological processes: trauma, malformation, inflammation, neoplasia and degeneration (see Table 5.1). Trauma may be external, e.g. road

Table 5.1 Summary of the causes of intracranial disorders.

Trauma	Road traffic accident
Malformation	FPV, griseofulvin
Inflammation	FIPV, FIV, *Toxoplasma gondii*, rabies, cryptococcus
Neoplasia	Meningioma, lymphosarcoma, astrocytoma, pituitary tumour
Degeneration	CIN, thiamine deficiency, renal failure, hepatic failure, hypocalcaemia, toxins

FIPV, Feline infectious peritonitis virus; FIV , feline immunodeficiency virus; FPV, feline panleucopenia virus; CIN, cerebral ischaemic necrosis.

traffic accident or internal, e.g. protruded discs. Inflammation is usually caused by an infectious agent, although immune-mediated processes are implicated in some cases. Neoplasia includes tumours arising from both the nervous system itself and from adjacent tissues which impinge on the nervous system. Degenerative neurological diseases may result from metabolic disorders, nutritional abnormalities, intoxication or vascular impairment. Idiopathic diseases are also placed in this category.

This is the first of two chapters describing the main diseases affecting the major divisions of the nervous system presented above.

INTRACRANIAL DISORDERS

The intracranial structures may be divided into three main functional areas, each of which when affected by a disease process produces a characteristic collection of signs. These areas are the forebrain, the cerebellum and the brainstem (Fig. 5.1).

Table 5.2 summarizes those signs which assist in localization of a disorder to the various regions of the brain.

TRAUMA

Head trauma can be sustained in a variety of ways, including road traffic accidents, dog bites and malicious wounding.

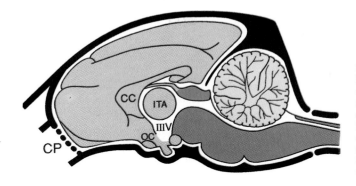

Fig. 5.1
Diagrammatic
representation of the
major functional
areas of the brain:
forebrain (pink),
cerebellum (yellow)
and brainstem (blue).
OC, Optic chiasm;
CP, cribriform plate;
IIIV, third ventricle;
CC, corpus callosum;
ITA, interthalamic
adhesion.

Table 5.2 Clinical signs associated with intracranial disease.

Forebrain	Behavioural abnormalities; aimless wandering, head pressing, aggression, depression Circling (usually toward the side of the lesion) Seizures Depression, stupor, coma Visual deficits usually contralateral to the side of a focal lesion Postural deficits Endocrine disturbances
Brainstem	Depression, stupor, coma Postural deficits (usually ipsilateral to the side of the lesion) Cranial nerve (CN) dysfunction; anisocoria (CN III); strabismus (CN III, IV, VI, VIII); facial paralysis (CN VII); masticatory muscle atrophy (CN V); head tilt, nystagmus, (vestibular disease) (CN VIII); dysphagia, laryngeal paralysis (CN IX, X)
Cerebellum	Ataxia, hypermetria, head and truncal sway, intention tremor, reduced/absent menace responses with intact vision Vestibular signs if the flocculonodular lobes are affected

Resulting neurological signs may range from depression to coma and depend on the degree of neuroaxonal and vascular damage. Penetrating calvarial wounds carry a high risk of haemorrhage and infection.

Elevated intracranial pressure (ICP) caused by progressive haemorrhage or oedema is a serious complication of many intracranial disease processes and should always be considered in animals with head trauma. Uncontrolled ICP elevations may lead to herniation of brain tissue underneath the falx cerebri, tentorium cerebelli or through the foramen magnum, all of which can be fatal. Therapy depends on the severity and progression of the injury and ranges from observation to intensive medical management. The full consequences of a traumatic episode may not be manifest at the time of the trauma. Haemorrhage, oedema and, possibly, infection may continue to evolve long after the injury, necessitating vigilance for at least 24–36 h (possibly several days) after the traumatic event.

Therapeutic considerations in animals are especially important in those with altered consciousness and include airway maintenance and oxygen supplementation, hyperventilation, judicious fluid therapy, corticosteroid therapy, hyperosmotic and diuretic agents. Much controversy exists over the use of corticosteroids in human head injury, some experimental literature suggesting that they may even potentiate intracranial pathology. Most veterinary neurologists still advocate their use and (although strict dose guidelines are not available) employ a regimen similar to that used for spinal trauma (Table 5.3). Mannitol, an osmotic diuretic, administered as a 20% or 25% solution at a dose of 1–2 g/kg over a 3–5 min period, should be considered in animals with severe (life threatening) signs or a rapidly deteriorating neurological status in whom elevated ICP is strongly suspected. Mannitol is probably best avoided in stable animals because of the possibility of producing rebound elevations in ICP. Frusemide 0.7 mg/kg given iv or im 15 min after the mannitol infusion may be used to enhance the duration of effect of the mannitol. Good renal function should be established before mannitol administration to avoid volume overload and pulmonary oedema. If blood gas analysis is feasible it should be performed in animals with altered consciousness to ensure adequate respiratory function as hypercapnia is a potent stimulus for cerebral vasodilation which raises intracranial pressure.

Table 5.3 High-dose corticosteroid therapy in the treatment of CNS injury

Spinal cord injury protocol	30 mg/kg MPSS intravenously as soon as possible after the injury
	15 mg/kg intravenously, 2 h after initial dose
	15 mg/kg intravenously, 6 h after initial dose
	2.5 mg/kg.h for the following 18 h

A single high dose of MPSS has also been demonstrated to be of benefit in a feline experimental head injury model

Head injury protocol	30 mg/kg MPSS intravenously within 8 h of the injury

Alternatives

1. Clinicians have also used prednisolone sodium succinate (Solu-Delta, Upjohn) in similar regimens

2. Dexamethasone 1–2 mg/kg iv. This dose has been used empirically for many years

MPSS, methyl prednisolone sodium succinate.

Post-traumatic seizures may be controlled with diazepam 0.5–1.0 mg/kg iv/im and/or phenobarbitone 2–6 mg/kg iv slowly. Pentobarbitone (5–15 mg/kg iv) may be used to effect for the treatment of refractory seizures. Anaesthesia of animals with traumatic intracranial injuries may be a high risk procedure as lowered vasomotor tone may further compromise intracranial blood flow. However, penetrating calvarial injuries and depression fractures carry significant risks of infection and haemorrhage and surgical intervention should be considered to lavage the wound, remove bone fragments or foreign material and stop haemorrhage.

MALFORMATION

The most common intracranial malformation is cerebellar hypoplasia caused by intrauterine or perinatal infection with feline panleucopenia virus (FPV) (Fig. 5.2). The virus causes cell destruction at the time of cerebellar development. The clinical signs of hypermetria, wide-based stance, whole-body and head sway and intention tremor of the head, become apparent at the

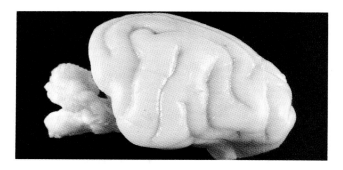

Fig. 5.2
Cerebellar hypoplasia in a kitten caused by feline panleucopenia virus.

onset of ambulation and are non-progressive. Menace responses are often absent although vision is normal (this is a common finding in many animals with diffuse cerebellar disease). Affected cats may make perfectly good pets. FPV infection may also be associated with inflammation of the ventricular system in the neonate which can interfere with the flow of CSF and lead to the development of hydrocephalus or hydranencephaly (Fig. 5.3).

The teratogenic effects of griseofulvin are well recognized and include a variety of fetal abnormalities, e.g. hydrocephalus, exencephaly and cyclopian deformities.

INFLAMMATION

Inflammatory disease is probably the largest category of feline intracranial disorders with infectious agents being the most common cause. The important infections are discussed here.

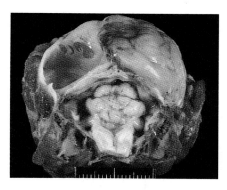

Fig. 5.3
Hydranencephaly and cerebellar hypoplasia in a kitten caused by feline panleucopenia virus.

Neurological signs are often multifocal and the disease may involve more than one organ system. Analysis of CSF typically reveals increases in the white blood cell population and the protein level. While confirming the presence of CNS pathology, unless an infectious agent is seen, these changes are often non-specific. All cats with suspected inflammatory neurological disease (and probably any undefined neurological disease) should be evaluated for feline leukaemia virus and feline immuno-deficiency virus infection.

Infection with the feline infectious peritonitis virus (FIPV) may produce a wide range of neurological signs and should be considered as a differential diagnosis in nearly all feline neuro-logical disorders. Neurological signs are most commonly associ-ated with the "dry" or non-effusive form of FIP although occasionally the "wet" or effusive form is incriminated. Single or multiple foci of pyogranulomatous inflammation are pro-duced which may involve any part of the CNS. Accordingly, the clinical signs can be diverse and they are usually progress-ive. They frequently include hind-limb paresis, nystagmus, and seizures. Pyrexia, depression and weight loss may also be apparent. Any age of cat may be affected, although FIP is usu-ally seen in animals under 3 years of age. Neurological disease associated with FIPV infection is often accompanied by ocular disease such as anterior uveitis (Fig. 5.4) or retinal vasculitis (Fig. 5.5) . Diagnostic features of FIPV infection include serum hypergammaglobulinaemia and raised cerebrospinal fluid (CSF) white cell count (mixed population of neutrophils and mononuclear cells) and protein levels. Serology is non-diagnos-tic because of the frequent incidence of false positive and false negative results. Definitive diagnosis is made on histopathol-ogy. Although the prognosis is poor, temporary improvements may be achieved with corticosteroid therapy.

Infection with *Toxoplasma gondii* may result in localized or multifocal, non-suppurative CNS inflammation. Although the cat is the definitive host for the toxoplasma organism, signs of systemic infection are uncommon. Affected cats usually show signs of pneumonia but occasionally signs of polioencephalo-myelitis may be present. The clinical signs, which are usually progressive, depend on the location and severity of the lesions and often include paresis/paralysis, seizures and behavioural changes. CSF analysis may reveal elevations in the white cell count and protein level. Neurological signs may also be

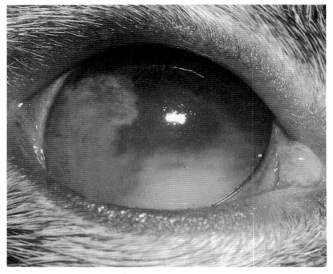

Fig. 5.4
Anterior uveitis
associated with feline
infectious peritonitis
virus infection.
(Photograph, M. G.
Davidson, North
Carolina State
University.)

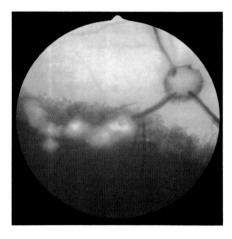

Fig. 5.5
Retinal vasculitis associated with feline infectious
peritonitis virus. (Photograph, M. G. Davidson,
North Carolina State University.)

accompanied by clinical and biochemical evidence of other organ involvement, e.g. uveitis, chorioretinitis (Fig. 5.6), pneumonia, hepatopathy (elevated liver enzymes) and myositis (elevated creatine kinase). Diagnosis relies on serological confirmation. IgG and IgM titres should be measured both acutely and after 2–4 weeks. IgM titres begin increasing 5–7 days post infection and elevated levels suggest acute infection. IgM titres return to normal after 3–12 weeks. Significant elevations in the

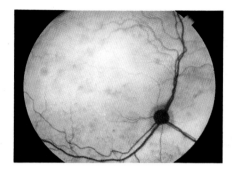

Fig. 5.6
Chorioretinitis associated with *Toxoplasma gondii* infection. (Photograph, M. G. Davidson, North Carolina State University.)

IgG titre are not detected for 10–14 days. A fourfold or greater titre elevation in a 3-week convalescent sample suggests recent infection. Antibodies may be detected in the CSF and aqueous humour in some cases. The prognosis is poor although improvement may be seen with clindamycin (25 mg/kg divided twice daily, by mouth, for 3 weeks) or potentiated sulphonamide therapy (e.g. trimethoprim sulfadiazine 30 mg/kg combined, twice daily, by mouth, for 3 weeks).

Rabies virus infection may typically produce signs of either depression and rapidly progressive paralysis ("dumb" form) or erratic, aggressive behaviour, wandering, salivation and tremors ("furious" form). Cats usually exhibit the furious form which often progresses to the dumb form. Definitive diagnosis is usually made post mortem by histopathology. Immunofluorescent testing of whisker follicles may provide antemortem confirmation in 25–50% of infected animals. From the time of development of neurologic signs, most animals will die within 3–5 days.

Feline polioencephalomyelitis is an uncommon disease of unknown aetiology reported in cats 3 months to 6 years of age. The inflammatory lesions predominantly affect the spinal cord producing progressive paresis and incoordination; however, the brain may become involved resulting in seizures.

Feline immunodeficiency virus (FIV) has been found in association with a variety of neurological diseases where its main pathogenic role is that of immunosuppression. The full significance of FIV as a neuropathogen is not yet known but recent investigations have identified primary CNS lesions which include perivascular cuffing, glial nodules and diffuse gliosis in subcortical nuclei.

In addition to its association with neoplasia, feline leukaemia virus infection has been observed in association with several poorly defined neurological syndromes e.g. urinary incontinence and anisocoria, but its primary role is probably similar to that of FIV, namely immunosuppression.

Cryptococcus neoformans is the commonest fungal infection of the CNS in cats. Following infection by inhalation the organism may invade the CNS haematogenously or by direct extension through the cribriform plate. Signs of focal or multifocal intracranial disease (Fig. 5.7) may occur which are often accompanied by respiratory, ocular or cutaneous disease. Diagnosis is made by cytological demonstration of the organisms, culture or serology. While the prognosis is poor, amphotericin B and ketoconazole have both been successfully used to treat affected cats.

Feline spongiform encephalopathy is a disease newly recognized in the wake of the bovine spongiform encephalopathy outbreak. Characterized by a variety of clinical signs that may include ataxia, behaviour change (timidity or aggression), hyperaesthesia, head nodding, muscle fasciculations, ptyalism, and jaw-champing, the condition is progressive and untreatable. Pathologic changes are seen throughout the CNS and include characteristic spongiform vacuolation of the grey matter, astrocytosis and microgliosis. The incidence and epi-

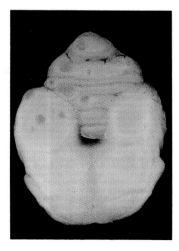

Fig. 5.7
Multifocal malacic areas in the brain parenchyma associated with *Cryptococcus neoformans* infection.

demiological significance of this disease is presently unknown. Diagnosis can only be confirmed by histopathology.

NEOPLASIA

Meningioma is the commonest intracranial neoplasm of cats, with a majority being found in the anterior fossa (rostral to the tentorium cerebelli) where they produce signs of forebrain disease. Affected cats are typically older (over 10 years) males. The neoplasm is slow-growing and may achieve a large size before clinical signs develop (Figs 5.8 and 5.9). Multiple meningiomas are not uncommon. Ante-mortem diagnosis is based on the history, clinical signs and computed tomography (CT) scanning or magnetic resonance imaging (MRI). Areas of mineralization within the tumour may occasionally be seen on plain radiography. Corticosteroid therapy may effect a temporary resolution of the signs but the long-term prognosis is poor without aggressive therapy. Surgical removal is the treatment of choice and offers an excellent prognosis; however, precise localization of the tumour using CT or MRI is required.

Other neoplasms affecting the brain include lymphosarcoma, ependymoma, pituitary adenoma and astrocytoma. The CNS is affected in only about 5–10% of cats with lymphosarcoma and the spinal cord is affected with a far greater frequency than the

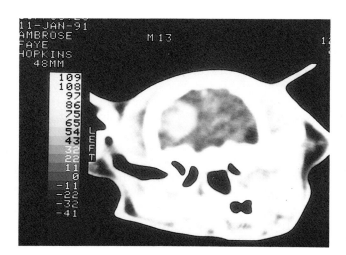

Fig. 5.8
Computed tomographic transverse section of the brain of a 12-year-old male cat demonstrating a large contrast-enhancing mass (meningioma) in the left parietal cortex.

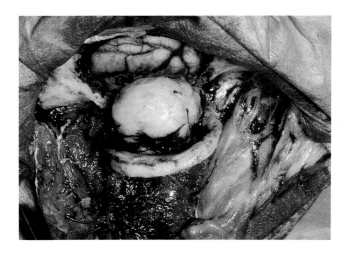

Fig. 5.9
The meningioma shown in Fig. 5.8 as seen at surgery. The neoplasm is approximately 2 cm in diameter.

brain. Pituitary tumours may give rise to endocrine disturbances such as hyperadrenocorticism and diabetes mellitus through oversecretion of adrenocorticotropic hormone and/or growth hormone.

DEGENERATION

Cerebral ischaemic necrosis (CIN), is an acute, unilateral, hypoxic insult to the forebrain. The aetiology is unknown but thrombosis and vasculitis of cerebral vessels have been observed in some cases. Adult cats of either sex may be affected. The clinical signs are acute in onset, usually non-progressive after the first 24 h and may include any combination of the signs characteristic of a forebrain disorder. Focal seizure activity may produce tonic/clonic muscle contractions on one side of the head or body. The severity of clinical signs is directly related to the size of the ischaemic area and infarction of two-thirds of one cerebral hemisphere may occur (Figs 5.10 and 5.11). Corticosteroids may be administered in doses equivalent to those used in intracranial and spinal trauma in order to suppress oedema formation around the ischaemic tissue. However, controversy also exists over the use of corticosteroids in vascular insults in human neurology. Diazepam and/or, phenobarbitone may be used for seizure control. The acute signs may

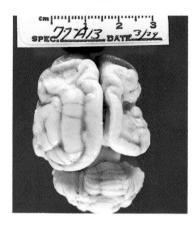

Fig. 5.10
Cerebral ischaemic necrosis. Note shrunken right cerebral hemisphere and left frontal cortex. (Photograph, A. De Lahunta, Cornell University.)

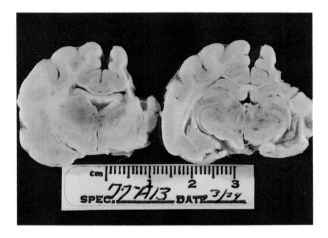

Fig. 5.11
Cerebral ischaemic necrosis. (Photograph, A. De Lahunta, Cornell University.)

regress in a few days and the prognosis is usually favourable although permanent deficits may be seen. The diagnosis is usually based on history and clinical signs. CSF analysis may reveal increases both in the protein level and the number of red and white cells.

Thiamine deficiency is primarily a brainstem disorder that occurs in cats fed either a raw fish diet high in thiaminase or an overcooked diet in which the thiamine has been denatured. Chronically anorexic cats are also susceptible to the disease particularly if they are systemically ill. Multifocal, malacic, haemorrhagic areas develop in the midbrain and brainstem nuclei. The clinical signs are often acute in onset and may include tetraparesis, vestibular dysfunction, pupillary abnormalities, ventral flexion of the neck and seizures. Treatment of thiamine deficiency includes corticosteroids to reduce oedema and 50–100 mg thiamine administered daily iv/im for up to 1 week, or until the cat is eating well. If treated early enough a response to therapy may be seen in a few days.

Metabolic abnormalities often result in signs referable to intracranial dysfunction. The clinical signs usually reflect diffuse forebrain dysfunction and are typically episodic in nature but may be persistent if the disease process is advanced.

Hepatic encephalopathy is uncommon in cats but may be secondary to congenital or acquired disorders. Clinical signs are characteristically episodic and include excessive salivation (ptyalism), behavioural change, depression and seizures. Typical biochemical abnormalities encountered include hypoalbuminaemia, low blood urea nitrogen, and hyperammonaemia. Liver enzyme concentrations are variably affected and may be normal. Pre- and 2-h post-prandial serum bile acid concentrations provide the most reliable way of demonstrating a functional hepatic abnormality. Nuclear scintigraphy and ultrasound may be used to demonstrate vascular abnormalities but the definitive diagnosis depends on radiographic demonstration of the anomalous vessel(s) using contrast portal venography (Fig. 5.12). Single, extrahepatic shunts are the commonest malformation found in cats and are often

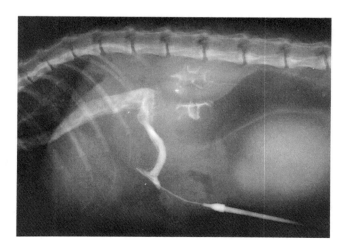

Fig. 5.12
Mesenteric portogram
demonstrating large,
single portosystemic
shunt.

amenable to surgical ligation. Diffuse hepatic disease or multiple shunts are usually managed medically. The goal of medical
therapy is to reduce the level of circulating toxins which
accumulate as a result of the hepatic insufficiency. Proteins are
thought to be the main source of these toxins following their
bacterial degradation in the large intestine. Ammonia and a
number of other toxins are generated in this way.

The diet should be of low protein (with a high biological
value), low fat and high carbohydrate content. Prescription diet
k/d (Hill's Pet Products) is formulated to fit these criteria. Oral
neomycin (20 mg/kg) four times daily by mouth and lactulose
(0.25–1.0 ml) one to three times daily by mouth are often used
in combination to reduce the population of bacteria in the large
intestine. Lactulose acidifies the large intestine resulting in trapping of the ammonium ion and acts as a laxative, decreasing
the time for absorption of toxins. The long-term prognosis with
medical management is poor.

Azotaemia in advanced renal failure may be associated with
profound depression, seizures (uraemic fits) and coma but this
is often a pre-terminal stage.

Hypoglycaemia is uncommon in the cat but may occur with
hepatic disorders, endotoxic shock, insulinoma, non-islet cell
neoplasms and iatrogenic insulin overdose.

Hypocalcaemia can occur in late pregnancy and up to 6
weeks post-partum. The characteristic signs of increased muscular tone, fasciculations and tremors, may be accompanied by
convulsions. Hypoparathyroidism has been reported as a cause
of hypocalcaemia in cats.

Lysosomal storage diseases are rare, inherited, cellular metabolic disorders of which several are now recognized in cats.
These include α-mannosidosis in Persian cats, mucopolysacch-
aridoses I and VI, sphingomyelinosis in Siamese cats, GM1 and
GM2-gangliosidoses, and globoid cell leucodystrophy. A specific enzyme deficiency results in accumulation of cellular metabolic products which subsequently disrupt normal cell function.
Many organs may be affected but nervous system dysfunction
is often first to become apparent. Signs are progressive and
often include depression, behavioural change, visual disturbances, seizures and ataxia with hypermetria. Hepatosplenome-
galy, skeletal abnormalities and ocular changes may also be
encountered. Young cats (less than 6 months old) are typically
affected. The defect is usually inherited in an autosomal reces-

sive fashion, so recognition of carriers and control of the trait is potentially simple.

Intoxication is not thought to be as common a problem in the cat as in the dog but the list of feline neurotoxins is continually increasing. Most toxins are accumulated by absorption through the skin, self-grooming of a contaminated hair coat or direct ingestion. The most commonly incriminated toxins are the organophosphates (OPs), carbamates and the chlorinated hydrocarbons used either excessively or inappropriately as parasiticides. The OPs and carbamates act as cholinesterase inhibitors, allowing excessive activity of acetylcholine at neuro-effector junctions. The clinical signs are usually acute, reflecting nicotinic and muscarinic receptor over-activity and include: salivation, vomiting, miosis, bradycardia, muscular tremors and convulsions. Treatment of intoxications should always include supportive fluid therapy. If the toxin has only recently been ingested, gastric lavage followed by the instillation of activated charcoal is indicated. Bathing the animal should be performed if a topical route of intoxication is apparent. Atropine (0.2 mg/kg with 25% of the dose given intravenously and the rest intramuscularly) is used to alleviate the muscarinic signs of OP and carbamate toxicity. The use of pralidoxime (2-PAM) is indicated in OP toxicity but not in carbamate toxicity. Chlorinated hydrocarbon toxicity is frequently associated with hyper-aesthesia and convulsions and also many of the signs of OP toxicity. Treatment is mainly supportive and symptomatic.

Prescription drugs may also result in signs of CNS disturbance if given excessively or inappropriately, or if they elicit an idiosyncratic drug reaction.

REFERENCES AND FURTHER READING

Center, S. A. & Hornbuckle, W. E. (1986) Congenital portosystemic shunts in cats. In *Current Veterinary Therapy IX: Small Animal Clinics* (ed. R. W. Kirk), pp. 825–830. Philadelphia, W. B. Saunders.

De Lahunta, A. (1983) *Veterinary Neuroanatomy and Clinical Neurology.* Philadelphia, W. B. Saunders.

Dow, S. W., Poss, M. L. & Hoover, E. A. (1990) Feline immunodeficiency virus infects cat central nervous system. *Proceedings of the American College of Veterinary Medicine 8th Annual Congress, Washington,* p. 1111.

Evans, R. J. (1989) Lysosomal storage diseases in dogs and cats. *Journal of Small Animal Practice* **30**, 144–150.

Greene, C. E. (1990) *Infectious Diseases of the Dog and Cat.* Philadelphia, W. B. Saunders.

Kornegay, J. N. (1981) Feline neurology. *Compendium on Continuing Education for the Practicing Veterinarian* **3**, 203–213.

Kornegay. J. N. (1989) Congenital cerebellar diseases of dogs and cats. *Current Veterinary Therapy.* pp. 838–841. Philadelphia, W. B. Saunders.

Lappin, M. R., Greene, C. E., Winston, S., Toll, S. L. & Epstein, M. E. (1989) Clinical feline toxoplasmosis. Serologic diagnosis and therapeutic management of 15 cases. *Journal of Veterinary Internal Medicine* **3**, 139–145.

Lawson, D. C., Burk, R. L. & Prata, R. G. (1984) Cerebral meningioma in the cat: Diagnosis and surgical treatment of ten cases. *Journal of the American Animal Hospital Association* **20**, 333–342.

Nafe, L. A. (1988) Selected neurotoxins. *Veterinary Clinics of North America: Small Animal Practice* **18**, 593–604.

Oliver, J. E. Jr., Hoerlein, B. F. & Mayhew, L. G. (1987) *Veterinary Neurology.* Philadelphia, W. B. Saunders.

Roberts, P. A., Pollay, M., Engles, C., Pendleton, B., Reynolds, E. & Stevens, F. A. (1987) Effect on intracranial pressure of furosemide with varying doses and administration rates of mannitol. *Journal of Neurosurgery* **66**, 440–446.

Shepherd, D. E. & De Lahunta, A. (1980) Central nervous system disease in the cat. *Compendium on Continuing Education for the Practicing Veterinarian* **2**, 306–311.

Skerritt, G. (1982) Brain disorders in dogs and cats. *In Practice* **4**, 81–86.

Zaki, F. A. & Nafe, L. A. (1980) Ischaemic encephalopathy and focal granulomatous meningoencephalitis in the cat. *Journal of Small Animal Practice* **21**, 429–438.

CHAPTER 6

Feline Neurology Part 2: Disorders of the Spinal Cord and Neuromuscular System

ANDREW HOPKINS

INTRODUCTION

The discussion that follows is based on the same approach to neurological disorders as found in Chapter 5. The term neuro-muscular system encompasses the peripheral nerve, neuro-muscular junction and muscle cell, disorders of which may be refered to as neuropathy, junctionopathy and myopathy, respectively. After localization of the lesion on the basis of the clinical signs, consideration is given to the signalment, history and the major categories of neurological disease allowing the formulation of a list of differential diagnoses and a diagnostic plan.

SPINAL CORD DISORDERS

Spinal cord disorders should be suspected in cats with weak (-paresis) or absent (-plegia) voluntary limb motor function in the absence of signs of brain dysfunction. This can be in one

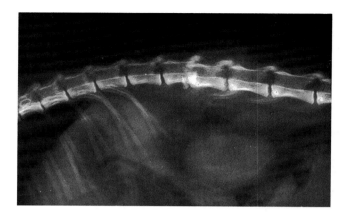

Fig. 6.1
Spinal fracture-
luxation with minor
displacement of the
vertebral bodies
apparent on the
lateral view.

limb (mono-), in both limbs on one side (hemi-), in both hindlimbs (para-), or in all four limbs (quadri-, tetra-). Disease processes are often limited to the spinal cord but the animal should
be examined for concomitant signs of dysfunction of the brain
and other body systems (especially the eyes) which may suggest
a multifocal disease process. An understanding of clinical
neuroanatomy is essential to localize and assess the severity of
the lesion. Following localization of a disease process to the
spinal cord, plain radiography and myelography are indicated
to define further the nature of the lesion. Lateral and ventrodorsal radiographs should always be taken when evaluating any
spinal cord disorder (Figs 6.1 and 6.2). Cerebrospinal fluid (CSF)

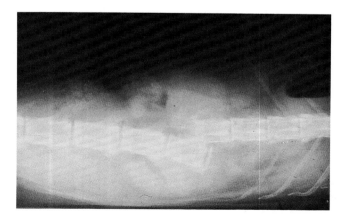

Fig. 6.2
Horizontal beam
ventrodorsal view of
the fracture in
Fig. 6.1
demonstrating gross
displacement and the
value of two views.

analysis is very important in the investigation of spinal cord diseases. If signs of multifocal disease are apparent (e.g. uveitis, nystagmus, seizures in conjunction with a definite spinal cord lesion) an infectious agent should be suspected and appropriate diagnostic testing for the organisms discussed in these chapters should be performed (see Table 6.1).

TRAUMA

Spinal cord injury may vary in severity from mild spinal cord contusion alone to grossly distracted spinal luxations or fracture luxations with severance of the spinal cord. Primary objectives are to identify the site and severity of cord injury and then to treat the lesion. The initial prognosis and treatment are based on the clinical signs and radiographic findings. Care must be taken to minimize movement of the cat during diagnostic procedures. Ventrodorsal views should be taken using a horizontal beam if spinal luxation is suspected, rather than rolling the animal on its back. Total functional spinal cord transection characterized by loss of voluntary motor function and absence of deep pain sensation always carries a very poor prognosis. Surgical stabilization should be considered if the site of injury appears unstable with the potential for deterioration of the neurological status. Cage rest and corticosteroid therapy is often a successful course of management for some spinal trauma cases. Extensive research has led to the use of high doses of corticosteroids for the treatment of spinal (and head) injuries (see Table 5.3).

Table 6.1 Summary of the causes of spinal cord disorders in the cat.

Trauma	Road traffic accident, disc protrusion, hypervitaminosis A
Malformation	Spina bifida
Inflammation	FIP, toxoplasma, polioencephalomyelitis, rabies, fungal infections
Neoplasia	Lymphosarcoma
Degeneration	Fibrocartilaginous embolism, thromboembolic myelopathy associated with cardiomyopathy

FIP, feline infectious peritonitis.

Table 6.2 Summary of the causes of peripheral nerve disorders in the cat.

Trauma	RTA, iatrogenic
Inflammation	Abscess, otitis media/interna, polyneuritis
Neoplasia	Primary nerve tumours (neurofibroma), infiltration (e.g. FeLV) or compression by adjacent tumour
Degeneration	Metabolic: (diabetes mellitus) Toxic: e.g. organophosphates, lead, aminoglycosides

RTA, Road traffic accident; FeLV, Feline leukaemia virus.

Administration of methyl prednisolone sodium succinate (MPSS) (Solu-Medrol, UpJohn) has been demonstrated to be beneficial to recovery of spinal cord injury in cats and humans (Hall, 1992).

Disc protrusions are a surprisingly common post-mortem finding in cats, but rarely cause clinical problems. If present, clinical signs are often a chronic progressive paraparesis (Fig. 6.3).

Hypervitaminosis A results in extensive bone proliferation around diarthrodial joints, especially in the spinal column. Neurological deficits may result from compression of the spinal cord.

MALFORMATION

The most common developmental abnormality of the feline spinal cord is spina bifida. This is a general term describing

Table 6.3 Summary of the causes of neuromuscular junction and muscle disorders in the cat.

Trauma	Traumatic myositis (RTA, bites)
Inflammation	Bacterial myositis following bite injury, immune-mediated polymyositis, myasthenia gravis
Degeneration	Metabolic: hypokalaemia, hypernatraemia, hypocalcaemia, aortic thromboembolism, botulism, tetanus, muscular dystrophy

RTA, Road traffic accident.

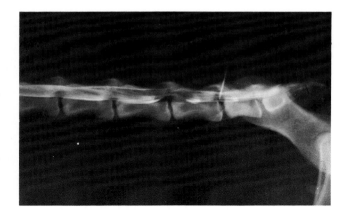

Fig. 6.3
Lateral view of a myelogram of a cat with chronic paraparesis caused by a disc protrusion.

several conditions involving varying degrees of failure of clos-ure of the vertebral arches alone or in conjunction with varying degrees of meningeal and/or spinal cord dysplasia (Fig. 6.4). Manx cats are the breed most commonly affected by this con-dition. Severely affected animals show signs of cauda equina dysfunction which may include a plantigrade hindlimb stance, faecal and urinary incontinence and secondary urinary tract infections.

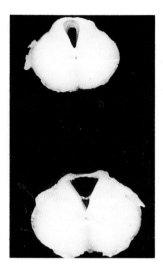

Fig. 6.4
Lumbar spinal cord of a Manx cat demonstrating syringomyelia and abnormal development of the dorsal horns (myelodysplasia). Courtesy of Dr D. J. Meuten, North Carolina State University.

INFLAMMATION

FIPV, toxoplasma, and polioencephalomyelitis have already been mentioned as causes of focal and multifocal CNS pathology. Often, signs of spinal cord dysfunction are accompanied by signs of intracranial and/or ocular involvement, but focal spinal lesions may occur.

Diagnostic findings suggestive of spinal cord inflammation include a normal myelogram or evidence of mild intramedullary swelling in conjunction with elevated levels of CSF protein and white blood cells. It is important to obtain CSF from the lumbar cistern in cats with focal spinal cord lesions, as samples obtained from the cerebellomedullary cistern may be normal because of the cranial to caudal direction of CSF flow.

The diagnostic procedures discussed in Part 1 for the investigation of inflammatory disease also apply here.

NEOPLASIA

Extradural lymphoma caused by feline leukaemia virus (FeLV) is the most common spinal tumour in cats (Fig. 6.5). Typically affecting young adult cats (3–4 years), most tumours are located in the thoracolumbar area and cause progressive pelvic limb weakness and pain. Clinical signs often develop over 3 days to 3 weeks. Other systemic signs of FeLV infection are often present.

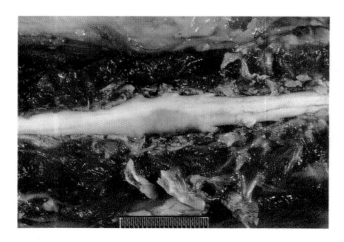

Fig. 6.5
Spinal
lymphosarcoma.

Lymphoblastic infiltration of the bone marrow is found in approximately 70% of cases and FeLV testing of the serum is positive in 85–100% of cases. Confirmation of the location and nature of the lesion requires myelography and possibly surgical or fluoroscopically guided needle biopsy. The long-term prognosis is poor but temporary remissions (4–5 months) may be obtained using combinations of corticosteroid, chemotherapy and radiation therapy.

FeLV has also been associated with proliferative bony lesions (osteochondromas) of the ribs, spine (Fig. 6.6), skull and limb bones. The lesions may be single or multiple and tend to cause pain and compress adjacent structures (e.g. spinal cord). Young adult cats are typically affected. Growth of the lesions is continuous and malignant transformation to osteosarcoma may occur. The prognosis is poor.

DEGENERATION

Fibrocartilaginous embolism has been reported in the cat, although it is rare. The signs of acute, focal, spinal cord dysfunction usually stabilize within 24 h. Therapy consists of cage rest and corticosteroids. The prognosis depends on the degree of functional impairment but if any recovery is to

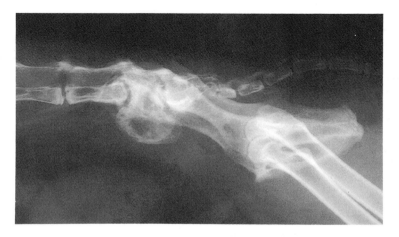

Fig. 6.6 Osteochondroma in a 1-year-old FeLV-positive male cat.

occur there will usually be signs in the 10–14 days following the initial episode.

Vascular occlusion and ischaemic myelopathy may occur in association with the thromboembolic syndrome seen in some cats with cardiomyopathy, however the arteries of the limbs (especially hindlimbs) are much more commonly involved in this condition.

NEUROMUSCULAR DISORDERS – PERIPHERAL NERVE DISORDERS

Peripheral nerve disorders most commonly involve one limb or nerve but several nerves may be affected in cases of multiple trauma and rare cases of diffuse inflammatory, degenerative or neoplastic diseases of the peripheral nervous system. Characteristic signs associated with peripheral nerve dysfunction include paresis or paralysis of the affected limb(s), muscle atrophy, hyporeflexia and hypotonia. These findings are often referred to as indicating a lower motor neurone (LMN) disorder. Sensory deficits are also common. Occasionally, a lesion may irritate a nerve and lead to the production of abnormal sensations (paraesthesias) in the sensory field supplied by that nerve. Selected cranial neuropathies are also covered in this section. On recognizing LMN signs it is important to consider the whole length of the nerve from its point of origin in the brainstem or spinal cord to the receptor or effector at its other end as the possible site of the disease process. Therefore LMN signs can occur with disease of the spinal cord or brainstem, peripheral receptor or effector as well as disease of the nerve trunk itself. This section is mainly concerned with disease of the nerve trunk. A detailed neurological examination with particular attention paid to peripheral neuroanatomy will often provide all the information required for diagnosis and prognosis. In more unusual conditions electrophysiological tests, muscle and nerve biopsy may be indicated.

TRAUMA

Trauma is the most common cause of peripheral nerve disorders in the cat and is usually associated with road traffic accidents. Nerves may be contused with no internal axonal disruption (neurapraxia), stretched with axonal disruption but with intact endoneurium (axonotmesis) or severed with complete disruption of the nerve (neurotmesis). A neurapraxic injury will usually recover with rest within a few days. Nerves suffering axonotmesis will usually recover following axonal regeneration which may take 1–2 months, depending on the level of the injury. Nerves usually regenerate at a rate of 1–2 mm per day. Up to 6 months may be required before a final assessment of degree of recovery may be made. Complete recovery of lacerated nerves is very unlikely but some return of function may occur with accurate surgical apposition of the severed ends of the nerve. The sciatic nerve is the most commonly injured, often in association with pelvic and/or femoral fractures.

Characteristic signs are seen in cats sustaining injury to the sacrocaudal spine. These may be grouped in order of increasing severity from having; (1) a paralysed tail alone, (2) a distended bladder that is difficult to express and which the cat continually strains to empty, (3) a distended bladder that cannot be expressed but which causes the animal no distress, and (4) a flaccid, atonic bladder with continual overflow and an areflexic anus. Radiographic abnormalities in these animals may be minimal. It is thought that the coccygeal, pudendal and pelvic nerves suffer traction injury and the extent to which the different nerves are affected determines the character and severity of the presenting syndome. With appropriate nursing the prognosis for the first two groups is good, the third poor and the last, grave. Cats that regain continence usually do so within a month. Tail paralysis may necessitate amputation.

The proliferative periarticular lesions of hypervitaminosis A may impinge on the spinal nerves as they leave the intervertebral foraminae, resulting in peripheral nerve dysfunction.

INFLAMMATION

Nerves may be affected at any point by an adjacent inflammatory process such as an abscess.

Primary inflammatory polyneuritides are rare but may be responsible for diffuse LMN dysfunction resulting in tetraparesis or tetraplegia.

Otitis media may cause a variety of neurological abnormalities. Ipsilateral facial paresis/paralysis and/or Horner's syn-

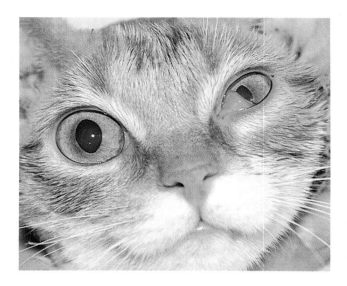

Fig. 6.7
Horner's syndrome in
a cat associated with
otitis media and
interna. Note miosis,
ptosis and protrusion
of the third eyelid.
(Photograph, N. J. H.
Sharp, North Carolina
State University.)

drome (Fig. 6.7) may result from involvement of the facial nerve
and post-ganglionic autonomic fibres, respectively, as they pass
very close to the middle ear cavity. Extension of the inflammatory process results in otitis interna and clinical signs of peripheral vestibular disease (head tilt (Fig. 6.8), nystagmus)
owing to disruption of the vestibular apparatus. Diagnosis of
otitis media requires thorough otoscopic examination, bulla

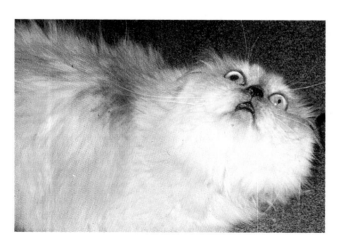

Fig. 6.8 Head tilt, a
hallmark of vestibular
disease. Central
(brainstem) and
peripheral
(vestibulocochlear
nerve and vestibular
apparatus) vestibular
disease should be
distinguished on the
basis of the
neurological signs.

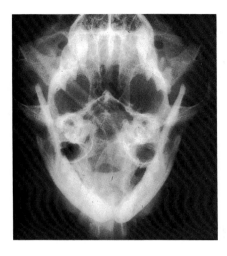

Fig. 6.9
Open mouth radiographic view of the tympanic bullae demonstrating sclerosis of the wall and increased opacity of the right bulla typical of otitis media.

radiography (Figs 6.9 and 6.10) (and computed tomography if available) and myringotomy. Therapy usually involves surgical drainage via a bulla osteotomy as antibiotic therapy alone is usually unsuccessful.

NEOPLASIA

Peripheral nerve dysfunction related to neoplasia is uncommon but nerves can be affected by primary neoplasms (e.g. neurofibroma), compressed by adjacent neoplasms or infiltrated

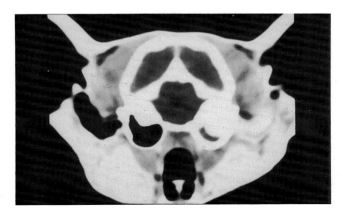

Fig. 6.10
Computed tomographic scan of the tympanic bullae of a cat with peripheral vestibular disease. A polyp was diagnosed at surgery.

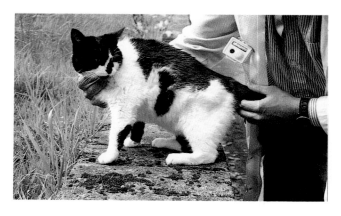

Fig. 6.11
Plantigrade stance in
a cat with diabetic
sciatic neuropathy.

by neoplastic cells (e.g. lymphoma). In addition to LMN signs, paraesthesias may cause the animal to lick and traumatize the skin of the appropriate sensory field.

DEGENERATION

Degenerative disorders of peripheral nerves are rare. Diabetic neuropathy may occur and is associated with a plantigrade hock posture (Fig. 6.11) which will often resolve following appropriate insulin therapy. Toxins such as heavy metals (e.g.

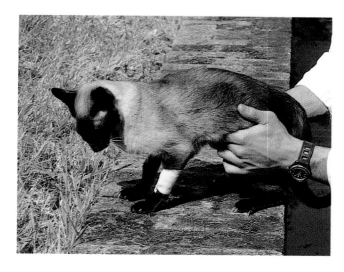

Fig. 6.12
Cervical ventroflexion
in a cat with
hypokalaemic
polymyopathy.

lead), organophosphates and chlorinated hydrocarbons can cause a variety of polyneuropathies.

Idiopathic nerve disorders are placed in this category, with probably the most well recognized being that of idiopathic peripheral vestibular disease. The syndrome is characterized by an acute onset of head tilt and nystagmus that may be so severe as to cause incessant rolling, crying and vomiting. The abnormality may be located in the vestibular apparatus or the vestibular nerves. Most cases are seen in the late summer and autumn. The aetiology is unknown. Resolution of clinical signs occurs over a period of 2–4 weeks. There is no specific therapy.

The aminoglycoside antibiotics (especially streptomycin) are known to cause peripheral vestibular disease in cats although their effects may be due to disruption of the vestibular apparatus rather than the vestibular nerves.

NEUROMUSCULAR DISORDERS – NEUROMUSCULAR JUNCTION AND MUSCLE DISORDERS

This group of disorders is relatively uncommon in the cat but encompasses one or two conditions that produce dramatic and characteristic clinical signs. Muscle diseases are associated with any combination of the following abnormalities: pain, pyrexia, generalized weakness that may be episodic, raised serum creatine kinase (CK) concentrations and abnormal muscle biopsy findings. Generalized muscular weakness results in exercise intolerance, a stiff gait and a marked ventroflexion of the neck. Evaluation and differentiation of the causes of muscle disease may require serological, biochemical, electrophysiological and muscle biopsy evaluation.

TRAUMA

Myositis frequently accompanies road traffic accidents and in severe cases the ensuing muscle damage may produce hyperkalaemia and myoglobinuria which should be considered in the management of trauma cases.

INFLAMMATION

Local or diffuse (polymyositis) inflammatory disorders may be encountered. Bite wounds and abscess formation are probably the most common cause of localized myositis and are usually resolved by drainage and appropriate antibiotic therapy. Polymyositis may be observed as a rare, idiopathic, suspected autoimmune disorder or in association with generalized toxoplasmosis.

Myasthenia gravis is included here because although the disease exhibits minimal inflammatory changes in the muscle tissue it results from an immune-mediated attack on the post-synaptic membrane. Clinical signs include exercise-induced muscular weakness, often manifest as progressive stiffness and collapse with cervical ventroflexion. Megaoesophagus may result in aspiration pneumonia and signs of respiratory distress. Thymomas have been associated with this condition in cats. Diagnosis is made on the basis of a response to intravenous edrophonium (0.05–0.1 mg/kg iv), electrodiagnostic testing and detection of antibody to the acetylcholine receptor.

DEGENERATION

Ischaemic neuromyopathy of the hindlimbs follows the thrombotic occlusion of the aortic trifurcation and produces very characteristic signs. Affected cats have a sudden onset of hindlimb paralysis associated with cold limbs, absent femoral pulses, cyanotic nail beds and, later, stiff painful hindlimb muscles. Paresis may be associated with a plantigrade stance. The patellar reflex is often intact while the withdrawal reflex and pain sensation are diminished. Occasionally, a thoracic limb may be affected. Serum CK levels are often dramatically elevated because of the hypoxic damage to the muscles. The condition is usually associated with cardiomyopathy (frequently hypertrophic) and the thrombus is thought to arise in the dilated atria. Vasoactive substances released by the thrombus cause vasoconstriction of the collateral circulation and subsequent profound ischaemia. The prognosis is guarded because of the underlying condition and the high risk of re-embolization. Recanalization may occur, accompanied by signs of improvement. In cats recovering from the initial episode survival times of up to 11 months have been reported. Aspirin or warfarin have been used to reduce the recurrence of clots. Appropriate steps should also be taken to manage the cardiac disease.

The organophosphate, fenthion, acts at cholinergic synapses similarly to other organophosphates but produces a different clinical picture in that skeletal muscle signs characterized by tremors and profound weakness predominate without parasympathetic dysfunction. Cervical ventroflexion is a common clinical sign. Treatment is the same as for other organophosphate intoxications. Diphenhydramine has been used to reverse the nicotinic signs.

Several, rare, muscular dystrophies have been reported in cats. These include feline hypertrophic muscular dystrophy, characterized by a stiff gait and muscle hypertrophy, Devon rex hereditary myopathy, characterized by muscle atrophy and cervical ventroflexion, and nemaline myopathy, characterized by weakness, muscle atrophy and trembling. Diagnosis is made on the basis of the clinical signs, electrodiagnostic testing and muscle biopsy.

Electrolyte disturbances may result in profound alterations in neuromuscular activity. Hypocalcaemia has already been mentioned in Chapter 5. Hypokalaemia is now well recognized as a cause of polymyopathy associated with generalized weakness, ventroflexion of the neck (Fig. 6.12) and raised CK levels. Hypernatraemia has also been reported as a cause of muscle weakness.

Cats are extremely resistant to tetanus, but botulism is occasionally reported and is seen as a diffuse LMN paresis or paralysis with no loss of sensation. Treatment is supportive and the prognosis is poor.

FURTHER READING

Braughler, J. M., Hall, E. D., Means, E. D., Waters, T. R. & Anderson, D. K. (1987) Evaluation of an intensive methyl prednisolone sodium succinate dosing regimen in experimental spinal cord injury. *Journal of Neurosurgery* **67**, 102–105.

Carpenter, J. L., Hoffman, E. P., Romanul, F. C. A., Kunkel, L. M., Rosales, R. K., Ma, N. S. F., Dasbach, J. J., Rae, J. F., Moore, F. M., McAfee, M. B. & Pearce, L. K. (1989) Feline muscular dystrophy with dystrophin deficiency. *American Journal of Pathology* **135**, 909–919.

Clemmons, R. M., Meyer, D. J., Sundlof, S. F., Rappaport, J. J., Fossler, M. E., Hubbell, J. & Dorsey-Lee, M. R. (1984) Correction of organophosphate-induced neuromuscular blockade by diphenhydramine. *American Journal of Veterinary Research* **45**, 1267–1269.

Deforest, M. E. & Basrur, P. K. (1979) Malformations and the Manx syndrome in cats. *Canadian Veterinary Journal* **20**, 304–314.

Delahunta, A. (1983) *Veterinary Neuroanatomy and Clinical Neurology.* Philadelphia, W. B. Saunders.

Griffiths, J. R. & Duncan, I. D. (1979) Ischaemic neuromyopathy in cats. *Veterinary Record* **104**, 518–522.

Hall, E. D. (1992) The neuroprotective pharmacology of methyl prednisolone. *Journal of Neurosurgery*, **76**, 13–22.

Joseph, R. J., Carrillo, J. M. & Lennon, V. A. (1988) Myasthenia gravis in the cat. *Journal of Veterinary Internal Medicine* **2**, 75–79.

Le Couteur, R. A. & Childs, G. A. (1989) Diseases of the spinal cord. In *Textbook of Veterinary Internal Medicine* (ed. Ettinger, S. J.), pp. 624–701. Philadelphia, W. B. Saunders.

Luttgen, P. J., Braund, K. G., Brawner, W. R. Jr. & Vandevelde, M. (1980) A retrospective study of twenty nine spinal tumours in the dog and cat. *Journal of Small Animal Practice* **21**, 213–226.

Moise, N. S. & Flanders, J. A. (1983) Micturition disorders in cats with sacro-caudal vertebral lesions. In *Current Veterinary Therapy: Small Animal Clinics* (ed. Kirk, R. W.), pp. 722–726. Philadelphia, W. B. Saunders.

Nafe, L. A. (1988) Selected neurotoxins. *Veterinary Clinics of North America: Small Animal Practice* **18**, 593–604.

Oliver, J. E., Hoerlein, B. F. & Mayhew, I. G. (1987) *Veterinary neurology.* Philadelphia, W. B. Saunders.

Pool, R. R. (1981) Osteochondromatosis. In *Pathophysiology in Small Animal Surgery* (ed. Bojrab, M. J.), pp. 641–649. Philadelphia, Lea & Febiger.

Spodnick, G. J., Berg, J., Moore, F. M. & Cotter, S. M. (1992) Spinal lymphoma in cats: 21 cases. *Journal of the American Veterinary Medical Association* **200**, 373–376.

Wheeler, S. J. (1989) Spinal tumours in cats. In *The Veterinary Annual* **29**, pp. 270–277. London, Wright.

CHAPTER 7

Cardiomyopathy

VIRGINIA LUIS FUENTES

INTRODUCTION

Acquired myocardial disease (or cardiomyopathy) is the most important cause of heart failure in cats. Bond and Fox (1984) estimated that up to 12% of cats have cardiomyopathy at post-mortem examination. Feline myocardial disease appears to be common but its presence may not be easily detected without careful investigation.

TYPES OF CARDIOMYOPATHY

Myocardial diseases can be classified by various criteria (see Table 7.1). No one system of classification adequately describes each condition and there is much overlap. The traditional classification of feline myocardial disease has been based on morphology (see Fig. 7.1).

Table 7.1 Classification schemes for feline cardiomyopathy.

Aetiology		
Primary	Idiopathic hypertrophic cardiomyopathy	
	Idiopathic dilated cardiomyopathy	
Secondary	Hyperthyroid cardiomyopathy	
	Hypertensive cardiomyopathy	
	Taurine deficiency	
	Acromegaly	
	Infiltrative neoplasia	
	Doxorubicin toxicity	
Cardiac morphology	Dilated cardiomyopathy	
	Hypertrophic cardiomyopathy	
	Restrictive/intermediate cardiomyopathy	
Cardiac function		
Systolic dysfunction	Dilated cardiomyopathy	
Diastolic dysfunction	Hypertrophic cardiomyopathy	
	Restrictive cardiomyopathy	
	Infiltrative neoplasia	

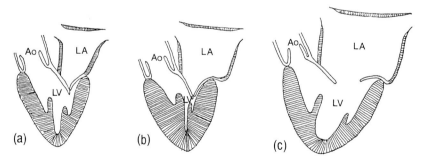

Fig. 7.1 Diagram of the left side of the feline heart. (a) Normal heart, (b) hypertrophic cardiomyopathy, (c) dilated cardiomyopathy. LA Left atrium, LV Left ventricle, Ao Aorta.

DILATED CARDIOMYOPATHY

Originally, dilated cardiomyopathy (DCM) was thought to be a primary myocardial disease in the cat. In 1987, it was discovered that the amino acid taurine played a vital role in myocardial function, and that dietary supplementation with taurine could reverse this form of cardiomyopathy in affected cats.

Because the levels of taurine in commercial diets have been increased, the incidence of DCM has been greatly reduced. DCM is now uncommon, although some cases still occur. It is likely that other factors are also involved in the aetiology of this condition, as in other species.

DCM is mainly seen in older cats and usually results in heart failure. Signs of right-sided heart failure often coexist with signs of left-sided heart failure. Poor contractile (systolic) function of the heart results in dilation of all the chambers. Affected cats usually respond poorly to symptomatic treatment although occasionally a cat might survive for as long as 6–12 months. Taurine therapy has radically altered the prognosis in DCM, as many cats now make a complete recovery after supplementation.

HYPERTROPHIC CARDIOMYOPATHY

Hypertrophic cardiomyopathy (HCM) is characterized by hypertrophy of the left ventricle, often with a reduced left ventricular diameter. Contractile function is good, but the left ventricle may be stiff and fail to relax properly, causing problems in ventricular filling (i.e. diastolic dysfunction). Hypertrophy of the ventricle is the normal response to increased ventricular pressure, but in idiopathic HCM there is no obvious cause of the hypertrophy. Left ventricular hypertrophy (LVH) also occurs as a response to systemic hypertension, with resulting cardiac changes that may be very similar to idiopathic HCM. Hyperthyroidism and excess growth hormone (acromegaly) also cause left ventricular hypertrophy. LVH may, therefore, be the end result of a number of different pathological conditions. Idiopathic HCM can be seen in any age, breed or sex of cat, but is most common in young to middle-aged male cats. In some cats the hypertrophy may be fairly localized rather than uniform; these cats may have a pressure gradient across the left ventricular outflow tract, and this variant is termed hypertrophic obstructive cardiomyopathy.

Affected cats may be asymptomatic for a period and then show sudden clinical deterioration with acute pulmonary oedema. Pleural effusions may also be seen but are less common. If the LVH is secondary to another systemic disorder, treatment of the primary problem may reverse many or all of the cardiac changes. In primary HCM, symptomatic treatment can alleviate signs for long periods in many cases.

INTERMEDIATE/RESTRICTIVE CARDIOMYOPATHY

Other categories of feline myocardial disease have been described, and have variously been termed "intermediate", "intergrade" and "restrictive". There is a lack of consensus over the exact definition of these terms, with some authors using all three terms interchangeably for cats with idiopathic myocardial disease which is neither hypertrophic nor dilated, and others reserving the term "restrictive" for cats with diastolic dysfunction associated with myocardial fibrosis. Certainly, there is much variation in the different forms of feline cardiomyopathy, with some cats developing signs of heart failure without an obviously hypertrophied or dilated heart. Many of these cats have very enlarged atria with normal left ventricular dimensions, suggesting abnormalities of ventricular filling, i.e. diastolic dysfunction. Some cats may also have subnormal systolic function. This group of myocardial conditions is particularly associated with dysrhythmias and aortic thromboembolism, although the usual reason for presentation is the development of congestive heart failure. The aetiology is usually obscure, although neoplastic or amyloid infiltration may very rarely result in similar effects.

TYPICAL HISTORY AND PRESENTING SIGNS

The most common presenting signs of feline cardiomyopathies are dyspnoea, anorexia, lethargy/weakness, hindlimb paresis, syncope and weight loss. Of these, respiratory difficulty is the most important, although many cats will show only vague and non-specific signs of illness. Anorexia and weakness are frequently present. The other major reason for presentation is limb paresis, caused by aortic thromboembolism. A less common presenting sign is vomiting. Coughing is rarely a sign of cardiac disease in cats.

The onset of acute pulmonary oedema or aortic thromboembolism may be dramatically sudden. Occasionally, the clinical signs are more insidious, with non-specific lethargy and inappetence. More frequently, the cat may be asymptomatic and signs of heart disease will be detected during routine examination or on presentation for another problem. A detailed history should be taken, including questions about diet.

CLINICAL EXAMINATION

Most cats with myocardial disease will show abnormalities that can be detected on physical examination and, in practice, the physical examination is the most valuable part of the investigation of cats with myocardial disease. A list of common physical findings is given in Table 7.2. A few asymptomatic cats may be normal on physical examination.

Cats with congestive failure usually present with dyspnoea. Those with severe dyspnoea may adopt open mouth breathing, with sternal recumbency and abducted elbows. Such cats are easily stressed and without careful handling will readily die.

Table 7.2 Common physical findings in feline myocardial disease.

Findings associated with cardiac disease
  Prominent apical impulse (especially hyperthyroidism)
  Systolic murmur
  Gallop sounds
  Dysrhythmias
  Palpable thyroid goitre (hyperthyroidism)
  Tachycardia (>240/min)/bradycardia (<150/min)
  Weak femoral pulse

Additional findings associated with congestive heart failure
  Dyspnoea/tachypnoea
  Hypothermia
  Pale mucous membranes/prolonged capillary refill time
  Cyanosis (with severe pulmonary oedema or pleural effusion)
  Distended jugular veins/(right-sided heart failure)
  Ventral dullness on percussion (pleural effusion)
  Muffled heart sounds (pleural effusion)
  Absent femoral pulse (aortic thromboembolism)
  Painful, paretic limbs (aortic thromboembolism)

Physical restraint in severely dyspnoeic cats should be kept to an absolute minimum.

Careful palpation of the neck may reveal the presence of a thyroid goitre in middle-aged or older cats. It is worth inspecting the jugular veins for signs of distension; this is a valuable clue to right-sided heart failure. It may be necessary to wet the coat in order to see the jugular veins if the coat is not to be clipped for venepuncture. Ascites is usually associated with non-cardiac conditions in cats but, when present with jugular distension, it can virtually be assumed that the aetiology is cardiac. Percussion of the chest may be useful in detecting a fluid line, which may be found with pleural effusions. Myocardial disease leading to congestive failure is one of the commoner causes of pleural effusions in cats. Pleural effusions are usually modified transudates and are pink-tinged or pale straw-coloured. Occasionally, effusions may be chylous.

Palpation of the chest is an undervalued part of the physical examination. Many cats with myocardial disease will have an exaggerated apex beat and in hyperthyroidism this can be dramatic. A reduced apical impulse will be found in a few cats with DCM, and also in cats with a pleural effusion. Dysrhythmias may also be detected by palpating the chest. Tachycardia is a frequent finding, but bradycardia may also be found (seldom seen in dogs with myocardial disease). Systolic murmurs are commonly heard on the left, but localization to a particular valve area may be difficult. Systolic murmurs may also be detected over the right hemithorax. Murmurs that are loudest over the sternum and right side of the chest may be associated with ventricular septal defects; these and other congenital defects may be present even in adult cats and can therefore be confused with myocardial disease. However, murmurs associated with myocardial disease are rarely loud enough to produce a thrill. It should be noted that some cats with myocardial disease may have no murmur at all, while others may have a variable murmur. Gallop sounds (where a third and/or fourth heart sound is present in addition to the first and second) are common findings. Gallop sounds may be heard only over a small area, so the chest should be auscultated carefully. The presence of gallop sounds is a fairly reliable indicator of myocardial disease.

The femoral pulse may be weak in DCM, or variable in dysrhythmias. One or both femoral pulses are usually absent in aortic thromboembolism. Occasionally, a forelimb may be affected, rather than one or both hindlimbs. Occlusion of an artery by an embolus is accompanied by release of vasoactive substances, which cause local vasoconstriction. The resulting ischaemic muscle damage may cause great pain and affected cats are often in obvious distress. Ischaemia of nerve and muscle results in a paretic limb with hard, cold and painful muscles. Other major arteries such as the renal arteries may also become involved, resulting in a spectrum of physical signs.

FURTHER INVESTIGATIONS

RADIOGRAPHY

Care should be taken if the cat is dyspnoeic. If a pleural effusion is strongly suspected from the physical findings, then thoraco-centesis should be performed before radiography. This will improve both the cat's chances of survival and the amount of information that can be obtained from the radiograph. If a cat becomes distressed easily a dorsoventral view may be more readily obtained than a lateral view. A second view may then be taken later, when the cat's respiratory function has improved. Ideally, the cat should be radiographed without sedation and with minimal physical restraint. With patience, a cat will some-times adopt sternal recumbency on an X-ray table without restraint of any kind.

Above all, it is imperative to keep the cat calm. When other means have failed, sedation may be necessary. Sedative com-binations used by the author for radiography in cats with car-diac disease are listed in Table 7.3, although all combinations using ketamine in uncompensated HCM are potentially hazard-ous.

Thoracic radiographs can demonstrate heart shape and size and also indicate volume overload in the pulmonary circulation. The normal feline heart occupies two rib spaces in width on a lateral view and two-thirds of the width of the chest on a dorsoventral view. In HCM, the heart may appear only slightly enlarged on a lateral view, but appear very broad on a dorso-ventral view, giving the so-called "valentine" shaped heart (Fig. 7.2). Genuine cardiomegaly may therefore be missed if only

Table 7.3 Sedative combinations for cats with cardiac disease.*

Acepromazine (0.1 mg/kg)
  + ketamine hydrochloride (5–7.5 mg/kg)
Midazolam (0.2 mg/kg)
  + ketamine hydrochloride (5–7.5 mg/kg)
Acepromazine (0.025–0.5 mg/kg)
  + midazolam (0.125–0.5 mg/kg)
  + ketamine hydrochloride (1–2.5 mg/kg)

* All combinations given intramuscularly.

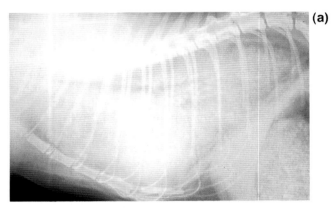

(a)

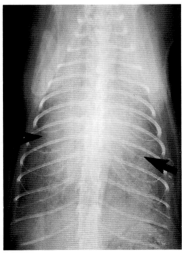

Fig. 7.2
Lateral and dorsoventral radiographs of the thorax of a 2-year-old neutered female Persian cat with HCM. (a) Severe generalized pulmonary oedema is present and, although the cardiac outline is unclear, it is possible to detect cardiac enlargement (arrows).

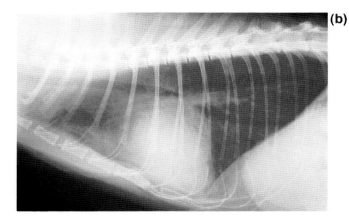

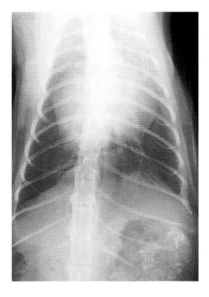

Fig. 7.2
(b) Radiographs taken after diuretic treatment 24 h
later show obvious cardiomegaly.

a lateral view is taken. In intermediate forms of cardiomyopathy
the atria may be obviously enlarged even on a lateral view. In
DCM the heart often shows general enlargement (see Fig. 7.3),
although it is not possible to distinguish the various forms of
cardiomyopathy by plain radiography alone.

(a)

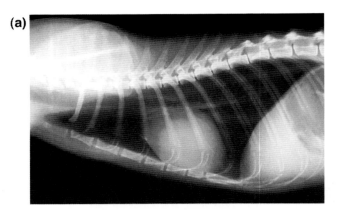

(b)

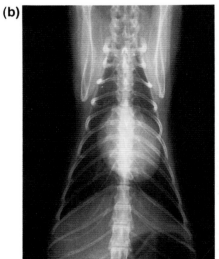

(c)

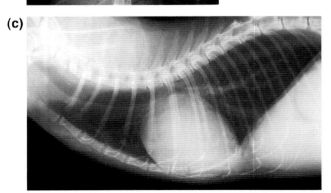

Fig. 7.3
Thoracic radiographs
of a 7-year-old
neutered female
domestic shorthaired
cat with dilated
cardiomyopathy
(DCM), showing
progression of
cardiomegaly. (a and
b) Mild cardiomegaly.
(c) one month later.

(d)

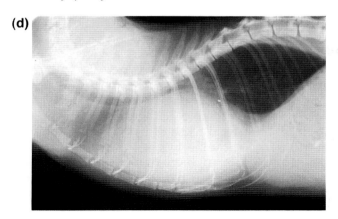

(e)

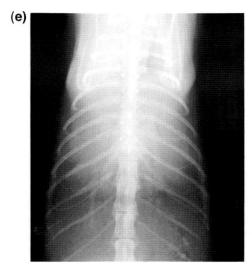

Fig. 7.3
(d and e) Three months later: gross cardiomegaly and congestive failure with probable pericardial effusion.

Radiographs are very useful for demonstrating signs of heart failure. Pulmonary oedema is often much patchier in cats than in dogs and may have a more lobar distribution (dogs frequently have either a perihilar or very generalized distribution). In congestive failure, the pulmonary vessels may be obviously distended. Pleural effusions that are not detected on percussion of the chest are usually readily demonstrated by radiography. However, small volumes may obscure all cardiovascular detail.

ELECTROCARDIOGRAPHY

In dyspnoeic cats, it may be necessary to delay recording an ECG if this causes distress, although placing the cat in a basket after attaching the leads can sometimes help. An ECG is essential, however, for the diagnosis of most dysrhythmias (see Table 7.4). The interpretation of feline ECGs can be complicated by the small complexes and rapid heart rates, but interpretation follows the same rules as for canine ECGs.

Waveform changes are also seen. Increased QRS voltages may indicate heart enlargement and are particularly common with hyperthyroidism. HCM can result in a partial bundle branch block (left anterior fascicular block) which gives deep S waves in leads II, III and aVF (see Fig. 7.4). This finding is fairly specific for HCM.

ECHOCARDIOGRAPHY

Echocardiography is the technique of choice for evaluating myocardial dysfunction, although its availability is limited in practice. It is a non-invasive, safe technique that provides valuable information (see Fig. 7.5).

Echocardiography allows the identification of the type of ventricular dysfunction, e.g. ventricular hypertrophy, or poor systolic function. This can be very helpful in deciding on rational treatment. Two-dimensional echocardiography can demonstrate: myocardial wall thickness, chamber dimensions, wall motility, presence of thrombi and congenital defects (such

Table 7.4 Commonly seen feline dysrhythmias.

Sinus tachycardia
Sinus bradycardia
Atrial premature complexes
Supraventricular tachycardia
Atrial fibrillation
Ventricular premature complexes
Ventricular tachycardia

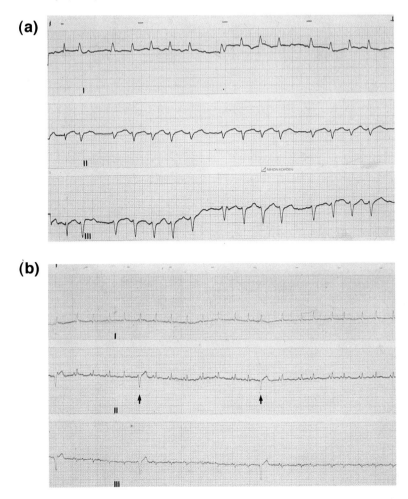

Fig. 7.4 (a) ECG showing leads I, II and III taken from a 2-year-old female Siamese cat with HCM. It shows atrial fibrillation, with no visible P waves and an irregular rhythm. This cat also had left anterior fascicular block (as shown here by a qR configuration in lead I and deep S waves in leads II and III). Paper speed = 50 mm/s; 1 cm = 1 mV. (b) ECG from a 6-year-old neutered male domestic short-haired cat with HCM showing leads I, II and III. Two ventricular premature complexes are shown (arrows). The other P-QRS complexes are normal in size and configuration. Paper speed = 25 mm/s; 1 cm = 1 mV.

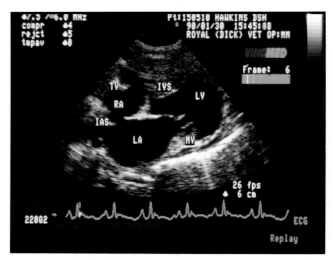

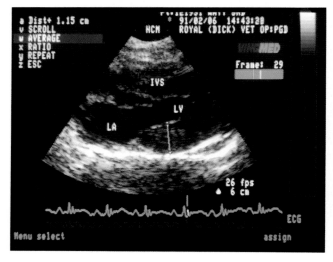

Fig. 7.5
Upper: Two-dimensional echocardiogram of an 11-year-old neutered female domestic shorthaired cat with DCM. It shows a dilated left atrium and left ventricle. Lower: similar view taken of a 4-year-old neutered male domestic shorthaired cat with HCM. The left ventricular free wall is greatly thickened (green line). Note the difference in ventricular wall thickness and diameter of the left ventricular lumen between the two cats. LA, left atrium; LV left ventricle; IAS, interatrial septum; IVS, interventricular septum; MV, mitral valve; TV, tricuspid valve; RA, right atrium.

as ventricular septal defect). Echocardiography will not usually indicate the precise aetiology of myocardial disease as, for example, the two-dimensional echocardiographic appearance of idiopathic HCM, hyperthyroid cardiomyopathy and hypertensive cardiomyopathy may be identical.

NON-SELECTIVE ANGIOGRAPHY

If echocardiography is unavailable, an alternative technique for distinguishing dilated from hypertrophic forms of myocardial disease is non-selective angiography. This is a relatively simple technique that can be performed in practice, although it is associated with more risks than echocardiography.

The cat's general condition must be stabilized before attempting angiography and plain thoracic radiographs should be obtained. The procedure may be performed under sedation, although it is usually carried out under general anaesthesia. One technique is to premedicate with one of the sedative combinations listed in Table 7.3, and then to induce anaesthesia with a mixture of halothane, oxygen and nitrous oxide by mask. The cat should be intubated and maintained with the gaseous mixture. An intravenous cannula should be placed in a jugular vein and a non-ionic soluble contrast agent containing at least 320 mg iodine/ml (e.g. Iohexol) at a dose of 0.75–1.5 ml/kg (maximum total dose 440 mg iodine/kg bodyweight) should be injected rapidly. It is possible to take multiple exposures following a single injection of contrast by pushing cassettes sequentially through a simple tunnel placed underneath the cat (Douglas *et al.*, 1987). The use of contrast media helps in the assessment of the thickness of the ventricular walls (see Fig. 7.6) and the degree of chamber dilation.

CLINICAL PATHOLOGY

Thyroxine levels (T4) should be measured in any middle-aged or ageing cat that presents with signs of cardiac disease, whether or not a thyroid goitre can be palpated. It is also sensible to check kidney function, as renal insufficiency can lead to systemic hypertension. Renal dysfunction may additionally be a contraindication for some cardiac drugs. Urine analysis is also important, as proteinuria may be the only abnormality in some cats with systemic hypertension caused by renal disease. It should be noted that renal thromboembolism can cause renal insufficiency.

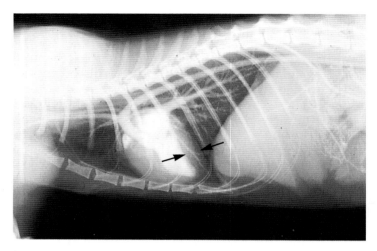

Fig. 7.6 Non-selective angiogram of a domestic shorthaired cat with HCM, showing opacification of the left atrium and left ventricle; note the thickness of the left ventricular wall (arrows) (picture, M. R. Oakley).

TREATMENT

If congestive failure is present, this may be treated before further investigations (see Table 7.5).

Life-threatening dyspnoea should be treated first and it may be necessary to attempt thoracocentesis before radiography. Sedation with acepromazine may be helpful if the cat is very

Table 7.5 Treatment protocols.

Pulmonary oedema	Administer oxygen
	Frusemide: initially 10 mg iv; repeated every 2–3 h if no improvement
	2% nitroglycerine ointment: $\frac{1}{8}$ inch every 8 h
	Cage rest
Pleural effusion	Thoracocentesis: aseptically prepare 7–8th intercostal space, infiltrate with local anaesthesia, attach butterfly cannula to three-way tap and withdraw fluid with syringe
	Continue as above

iv, Intravenously.

distressed. Thromboembolism requires treatment (see Table 7.6) before further investigations can be carried out to ascertain the precise form of cardiomyopathy. After initial drainage, moderate pleural effusions may be managed by diuretic therapy. Severe effusions may require placement of a chest drain.

TREATMENT OF THROMBOEMBOLISM

Pain relief is probably the first priority with many cases of thromboembolism, but concurrent signs of congestive failure should not be neglected. Cardiac decompensation is the most common cause of death in acute cases of thromboembolism. Sodium heparin may be given to prevent extension of the existing thrombus. Surgical embolectomy is contraindicated, as the benefits do not outweigh the risks. Drug therapy for lysis of thrombi is expensive and has been associated with increased mortality. Local vasoconstriction may be reduced (and local perfusion thus improved) by the use of acepromazine.

If the cat can be kept comfortable and signs of congestive failure controlled, the pulse will often return within a few days. Some cats will make a complete recovery; others may develop extensive skin and muscle necrosis or have permanent neurological deficits. Subsequent maintenance with aspirin may help to prevent further thromboembolism, although this has not been proven. Sadly, many cats experience further bouts of thromboembolism after recovery from the first episode.

Table 7.6 Treatment for thromboembolism.

Analgesia (morphine 0.1 mg/kg sc)

Prevent extension of thrombus (sodium heparin 200 iu/kg every 8 h for 2–3 days)

Promote vasodilation (acepromazine 0.1 mg/kg sc)

Treat congestive failure (see Table 7.5)

Keep warm, cage rest

Maintain on aspirin (20–25 mg/kg twice a week)

sc, Subcutaneously.

SPECIFIC TREATMENT

The initial approach should be towards the control of congestive failure signs with diuretics and, if required, thoracocentesis and vasodilators. Thereafter, more specific therapy can be directed at the underlying primary problem, or at least towards the specific functional abnormality (see Table 7.7). Hyperthyroid cardiomyopathy, for example, may be completely reversible if the underlying hyperthyroidism is corrected.

It is safer to avoid using drugs such as digoxin and propranolol if the underlying cause of congestive failure is not apparent. Frusemide is the only cardiac drug that is licensed for use in cats and is the mainstay of treatment of congestive heart failure. The vasodilator enalapril (an angiotensin converting enzyme (ACE) inhibitor) may be used to good effect if signs of congestive failure persist. There are some theoretical arguments against the use of ACE inhibitors in hypertrophic obstructive cardiomyopathy but, in practice, ACE inhibitors often seem effective in controlling congestive signs.

Table 7.7 Treatment for systolic and diastolic dysfunctions.

Systolic dysfunction	Diastolic dysfunction
Correct the diet	Slow heart rate/improve relaxation: Propranolol 2.5–5 mg PO every 8–12 h; or diltiazem 7.5 mg PO every 12 h (difficult to divide)
Administer taurine (250 mg bid)	
Supportive therapy until improvement: Frusemide 10 mg PO every 12–24 h, nitroglycerine ointment $\frac{1}{8}$ inch every 12 h, enalapril 0.5 mg/kg PO every 12–24 h, digoxin 0.0625 mg, half a tablet PO every 6–48 h	Supportive therapy for congestive failure: Frusemide 10 mg PO every 12–24 h plus enalapril 0.5 mg/kg PO every 12–24 h if congestive signs persist

bid, Twice daily; PO, by mouth.

PROGNOSIS

The prognosis varies greatly according to the type of myocardial disease and the treatment. Primary HCM may respond well to treatment and affected cats can remain asymptomatic for long periods. However, some cats will develop thromboembolism and sudden death is not uncommon. As already stated, HCM secondary to hyperthyroidism usually responds well to thyroidectomy or thyrotoxic drug treatment, but the management of HCM secondary to hypertension may be more difficult. There are no studies to date documenting the best treatment for systemic hypertension in cats because it is so difficult to monitor blood pressure. DCM usually responds well to taurine supplementation, although cats that fail to respond have a poor prognosis.

CONCLUSION

Feline myocardial disease is common in clinical practice, but may be missed without careful examination. Cats with suspected heart disease should be thoroughly investigated, as treatment of specific underlying causes can lead to complete resolution of myocardial dysfunction. In primary myocardial disease, knowledge of the underlying pathophysiology can help in selecting specific drug therapy. Treatment of feline myocardial disease can often be surprisingly rewarding.

REFERENCES AND FURTHER READING

Atkins, C. E., Gallo, A. M., Kurzman, I. D. & Cowan, P. (1992) Risk factors, clinical signs and survival in cats with a clinical diagnosis of idiopathic hypertrophic cardiomyopathy: 74 cases (1985–1989). *Journal of the American Veterinary Medical Association* **201**, 613–618.

Bonagura, J. D. (1989) Cardiovascular diseases. In *The Cat: Diseases and Clinical Management* (ed. Sherding, R. G.), pp. 649–753. New York, Churchill Livingstone.

Bond, B. R. (1986) Hyperthyroid heart disease in cats. In *Current Veterinary Therapy IX* (ed. Kirk, R. W.), pp. 399–402. Philadelphia, W. B. Saunders.

Bond, B. R. & Fox, P. R. (1984) Advances in feline cardiomyopathy. *Veterinary Clinics of North America* **14**, 1021–1038.

Douglas, S. W., Herrtage, M. E. & Williamson, H. D. (1987) Angiography. In *Principles of Veterinary Radiography*, 4th edn, pp. 270–273. London, Baillière Tindall.

Flanders, J. A. (1986) Feline aortic thromboembolism. *Compendium on Continuing Education for the Practicing Veterinarian* **8**, 473–484.

Fox, P. R. (ed) (1988) Feline myocardial disease. In *Canine and Feline Cardiology* pp. 435–466. New York, Churchill Livingstone.

Harpster, N. K. (1986) The cardiovascular system. In *Diseases of the Cat: Medicine and Surgery* (ed. Holzworth, J.), pp. 820–933. Philadelphia, W. B. Saunders.

Kobayashi, D. L., Peterson, M. E., Graves, T. K., Lesser, M. & Nichols, C. E. (1990) Hypertension in cats with chronic renal failure or hyperthyroidism. *Journal of Veterinary Internal Medicine* **4**, 58–62.

Peterson, M. E., Taylor, S., Greco, D. S., Nelson, R. W., Randolph, J. F., Foodman, M. S., Moroff, S. D., Morrison, S. A. & Lothrop, C. D. (1990) Acromegaly in 14 cats. *Journal of Veterinary Internal Medicine* **4**, 192–201.

Pion, P. D. & Kittleson, M. D. (1989) Therapy for feline aortic thromboembolism. In *Current Veterinary Therapy X* (ed. Kirk, R. W.), pp. 295–302. Philadelphia, W. B. Saunders.

Pion, P. D., Kittleson, M. D. & Rogers, Q. R. (1989) Cardiomyopathy in the cat and its relation to taurine deficiency. In *Current Veterinary Therapy X* (ed. Kirk, R. W.), pp. 251–262. Philadelphia, W. B. Saunders.

CHAPTER 8

Helminths

MAGGIE FISHER

INTRODUCTION

The estimated population of domestic cats in the UK is 7.2 million. The majority of those that have access to the outdoor environment are likely to be frequently exposed to helminth infection, particularly in areas of high domestic or feral cat population density. Places used for defecation are often shared by a number of cats over a long period, which may lead to the contamination of cats' paws with infective eggs as they bury their faeces. While the dog population is, in general, more controlled, cats continue to live an independent existence. Many hunt and eat the invertebrates, birds and small mammals that act as intermediate or transport hosts for helminth parasites.

This does not mean that cats kept in controlled conditions, such as those in breeding colonies and indoor cats in multi-cat domestic households, are not likely to be infected with helminths. Given the right conditions, particularly lack of hygiene and infrequent cleaning of litter trays, worm infections may occur and may be transmitted.

WHY WORRY?

Most owners find the idea of their pet being infected with
worms quite repugnant, particularly when the evidence crawls
or is vomited into view. Some cat helminths have zoonotic
potential: *Dipylidium caninum* infection in man has been
recorded, albeit rarely. *Toxocara cati* larvae have occasionally
been identified in cases of larval migrans in man, though *T.
canis* larvae are usually responsible. Helminth infection may
cause severe illness in the feline host, although low worm bur-
dens are normally inapparent. A heavy *T. cati* infection in kittens will result in poor growth and inefficient food conversion.
Occasionally deaths will occur due to intestinal obstruction.

CESTODES

There are two cestodes or tapeworms that occur in domestic
cats in the UK – *D. caninum* and *Taenia taeniaeformis. D. caninum*
is the most common and it is generally believed that the same
species occurs in both cats and dogs. In a survey of 1149 London
cats, 1.1% of domestic and 20.0% of feral cats were found to be
infected with *D. caninum*, while 1.1% of domestic and 6.8% of
feral cats were found to harbour *T. taeniaeformis.* The figures for
infection in domestic cats were probably underestimated as they
were based on the presence of eggs or segments in faecal
samples and these are not consistently present in cases of cestode infection.

SMALL INTESTINE – *DIPYLIDIUM CANINUM*

The adult tapeworm has a scolex with a protrusible armed rostellum and is between 20 and 50 cm long. There may be many
worms present in an animal, apparently without deleterious
effect. Mature proglottids, each containing groups of eggs
enclosed in egg packets, break off the caudal end of the worm
and are passed in the faeces. The proglottids are motile when
first passed and may be recognized by their white semilucent

"rice grain" appearance (see Fig. 8.1). Each segment has one genital pore, seen as an inversion, on each side.

(a)

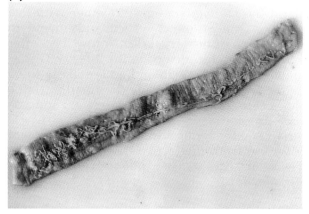

(b)

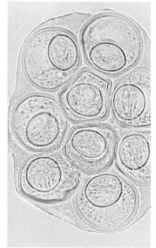

(c)

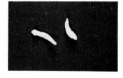

Fig. 8.1

(a) Adult *Dipylidium caninum in situ.* (b) Group of *D. caninum* eggs, each approximately 30 μm in diameter, enclosed in an egg packet. (c) *D. caninum* proglottid, approximately 1 cm in length, showing "rice grain" appearance and the genital pore on each side.

Life cycle

The flea, primarily *Ctenocephalides felis*, acts as the intermediate host in the cat. Some *Dipylidium* species segments fall to the ground in places heavily contaminated with flea eggs. Flea larvae may then ingest the *D. caninum* eggs, together with flea faeces and other debris. One or more cysticercoids begin to develop within the abdomen of the larval flea. A few days after emerging from the pupa, the adult flea contains infective meta-cestodes. Such fleas tend to be sluggish and so are likely to be ingested by the cat as it grooms. Once inside the small intestine of the cat, the scolex everts, attaches to the intestinal mucosa and starts to produce proglottids.

The prepatent period is only about 3 weeks so it is important to differentiate reinfection from ineffective treatment of a previous infection. There appears to be little or no acquired immunity following infection.

Control of *Dipylidium* species infection

It is important to control both fleas and tapeworms in order to eliminate infection with *Dipylidium* species. Flea control should be targeted at control of the adult flea on the cat (1, 2) and control of the immature stages in the environment (3, 4) by:

(1)   Insecticidal treatment
(2)   Regular grooming using a very fine-toothed comb
(3)   Hoovering and cleaning of the cat's indoor environment
(4)   Either environmental spray containing insecticide or insecticide plus larval growth inhibitor or lufenuron (Program, Ciba Animal Health) treatment of cat.

The cat should be treated at the same time with an appropriate cestocide.

SMALL INTESTINE – *TAENIA TAENIAEFORMIS*

T. taeniaeformis is similar in appearance to *Taenia* species that occur in other animals (see Fig. 8.2), the scolex bears four suckers and an armed rostellum with two rows of hooks. The adult

(a)

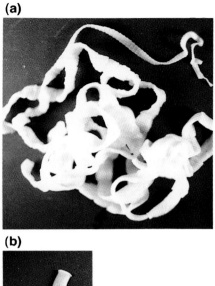

(b)

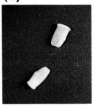

(c)

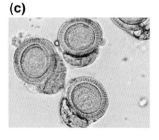

Fig. 8.2
(a) Adult *Taenia taeniaeformis.* (b) Mature *T. taeniaeformis* proglottid, approximately 1 cm long, with single genital pore. (c) Typical taeniid egg (approximately 35 μm diameter).

worm is about 60 cm long and attaches to the intestinal mucosa by means of the hooks and suckers. The mature proglottids have a rectangular shape (longer than they are broad) with one genital pore. They are more opaque than a segment from *Dipylidium* species.

The gravid proglottid is passed in the faeces and then disintegrates in the environment, releasing the eggs. Rodents, which act as intermediate hosts, eat the eggs which develop to form pea-sized nodular strobilicerci in the animal's liver. The cat is infected when it, in turn, ingests the rodent containing the infective metacestode.

NEMATODES

STOMACH – *OLLULANUS TRICUSPIS*

Ollulanus tricuspis is such a small (approximately 1 mm long) worm that it is usually overlooked, thus there is little information on the incidence of infection. The adult worms live in the gastric mucosa and the females produce larvae capable of maturing to adults inside that same host. Transmission is thought to occur via vomit containing the third-stage larva. *Ollulanus* species has been reported as the cause of a high incidence of vomiting and diarrhoea in a cat colony. Diagnosis is based on examination of either vomit or post-mortem histology for the adult worms or larvae. Benzimidazole treatment may be helpful, but specific dose schedules are not known.

SMALL INTESTINE – *TOXOCARA CATI* AND *TOXASCARIS LEONINA*

T. cati (Fig. 8.3) and *Toxascaris leonina* have the typical appearance of ascarids – thick, fleshy worms about 12 cm long. The adult worms can be differentiated by the appearance of their cervical alae: those of *T. cati* have an arrow-headed shape

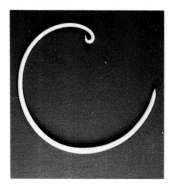

Fig. 8.3
Adult *Toxocara cati*, approximately 8 cm long.

while those of *T. leonina* have a more tapered or lanceolate appearance (see Fig. 8.4). Studies have shown approximately 28% (range 3.9–49.3%) of cats in the UK to be infected with *T. cati*, with the highest incidence in feral and young cats. *T. leonina* is much less prevalent, present in 0–5.5% of cats.

Life cycle

Cats may be infected with *T. cati* by: ingestion of an egg containing a second-stage larva; ingestion of a paratenic host such as a rodent, bird or mollusc; or transmammary infection.

Unlike *T. canis* infection, there is no transplacental transfer. Second-stage larvae contained within eggs that are ingested undergo hepatotracheal migration before returning to the intestine as third-stage larvae to complete their development in the intestinal mucosa. The prepatent period is about 8 weeks. Following infection by larvae ingested within a paratenic host or in milk, the worms develop in the intestine without further migration. The prepatent period is subsequently only 6 weeks.

Patent infections may be seen in kittens aged 6 weeks or more, or as a mixed infection with *T. leonina* in older cats.

A heavy burden will lead to a pot-bellied appearance, diarrhoea, vomiting and "poor doing".

Infection with *T. leonina* occurs by ingestion of either an egg containing a second-stage larva or an intermediate host, such

(a)   **(b)**

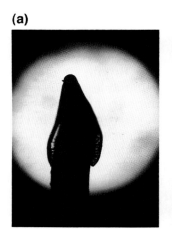 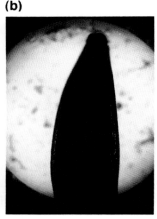

Fig. 8.4
(a) The anterior region of an adult *Toxocara cati*, showing the arrow-shaped cervical alae. (b) The anterior region of an adult *Toxascaris leonina*, showing the lanceolate cervical alae.

as a mouse carrying third-stage larvae. Whatever the source of infection, development occurs in the intestine with no migratory stage. The prepatent period is about 11 weeks and infection is seen in the adolescent and adult cat.

Diagnosis

Diagnosis of patent *T. cati* or *T. leonina* infection is based on demonstration of eggs in the faeces by McMaster or other flotation techniques. Fresh *T. cati* eggs are dark, subcircular and have a thick, pitted shell while *T. leonina* eggs have a lighter appearance and a thick, smooth shell.

Treatment

Piperazine is commonly used to treat roundworm infections in kittens. Before using piperazine, care should be taken to assess the bodyweight accurately. There have been a number of reports over the past few years of ataxia following overdosage in cats. A benzimidazole such as fenbendazole (Panacur, Hoechst) is likely to be more consistently effective. Panacur is available in suspension or granule form. The granules are often convenient as they can be mixed with food by owners who are unable to restrain their cats.

SMALL INTESTINE – HOOKWORM

Hookworm eggs have been recorded, albeit uncommonly, in faecal samples from cats, usually feral, in Britain. It remains unclear whether such infections are attributable to *Uncinaria stenocephala*, the hookworm that also commonly affects dogs in the UK, or *Ancylostoma tubaeforme*, the hookworm that infects cats all over the world. The hookworm life cycle is direct. Cats are infected by ingesting infective larvae that have developed from eggs passed in the faeces. *Ancylostoma* species larvae may also infect percutaneously. Hookworm infections have not been associated with clinical signs in the UK.

Diagnosis is based on demonstration of typical strongyle-type eggs in the faeces by a McMaster or other flotation technique.

LUNGS – *AELUROSTRONGYLUS ABSTRUSUS*

The adult worms of *Aelurostrongylus abstrusus* are slender and about 1 cm long. They are usually embedded within the lung parenchyma so are difficult to recover intact (see Fig. 8.5). Hamilton (1963) found that 12 out of 125 (9.3%) cats were infected during a post-mortem survey.

Life cycle

The eggs produced by the female worm have already hatched into first-stage larvae by the time that they are coughed up, swallowed and pass out in the faeces. The larvae penetrate the foot of a slug or snail and develop to third-stage larvae within the intermediate host. A cat is infected when it ingests an infected mollusc, or a rodent or bird that is acting as a paratenic host. From the cat's intestine the larvae travel to the lungs via the lymphatic system or bloodstream.

Pathology

Greyish foci are grossly visible throughout the substance of the lungs. These may be small, discrete nodules composed of

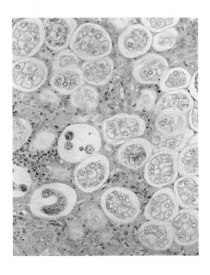

Fig. 8.5
Section through a cat's lung, showing adult *Aelurostrongylus* species worms surrounded by inflammatory cells.

inflammatory cells, adult worms, eggs and larvae or may be much larger coalescing lesions with caseous centres. Hypertrophy of the muscles of the bronchioles, alveolar ducts and media of the pulmonary arteries occurs.

Clinical signs

Infection is usually asymptomatic or associated with no more than a slight cough that increases on exercise, possibly with sneezing and a mucoid nasal discharge. In most animals clinical signs are transient and improvement is associated with resolution of the lung lesions. Occasionally, more severe symptoms will occur in an individual, including dyspnoea and coughing. In such cases treatment may be necessary.

Diagnosis

Diagnosis is based on the presence of first-stage larvae in samples of tracheal mucus or the demonstration of the larvae in faeces by faecal smear or by use of the Baermann technique. The larvae may be recognized by their S-shaped tails. The presence of eosinophils in the tracheal mucus, an eosinophilia and neutrophilia, together with small patches of opacity throughout the lung field on radiography, are non-specific but may assist the diagnosis.

OTHER NEMATODE INFECTIONS

Very rarely *Capillaria aerophila* infection may occur in the trachea or bronchi of cats and *Capillaria plica* may affect the bladder. Diagnosis is based on demonstration of eggs with bipolar plugs in the faeces or the urine, respectively.

ANTHELMINTICS AND WORM CONTROL

TREATMENT OF CESTODE INFECTIONS

The anthelmintics currently available for use against tapeworm infections in cats are either specific cestocides or products with a broad spectrum of activity (Table 8.1). All are available as oral preparations, most in tablet form, although fenbendazole (Panacur, Hoechst) is available in a granular formulation that can be readily mixed with food. Praziquantel (Droncit, Bayer) is also marketed in a form suitable for subcutaneous or intramuscular injection. Dilution of Droncit with even minute amounts of water (as may happen, for example, when reusing a syringe that has not been totally dried) must be avoided as this may cause a stinging sensation at the infection site and/or, decreased cestocidal activity.

No prior starvation is necessary with any of the products, and owners may find it easiest to administer tablet and granular preparations mixed in with food. The benzimidazoles are likely to be more effective when given by a divided dose schedule rather than as a single large dose; therefore, the divided dose regimen is recommended where the data sheet suggests both alternatives. Both praziquantel and the benzimidazoles have a wide safety margin between the therapeutic dose and the dose where toxic signs may be seen. Tapeworms are often digested after treatment and so frequently no evidence of their expulsion is seen in the faeces.

TREATMENT OF NEMATODE INFECTIONS

Anthelmintics available for the treatment of nematode infections are shown in Table 8.1. The only product with a data sheet recommendation for treatment of *Aelurostrongylus abstrusus* infection is fenbendazole (Panacur, Hoechst) at a dose rate of 50 mg/kg.day for 3 days.

Table 8.1 Anthelmintics for use in the cat.

Anthelmintic	Product name	Company	Toxocara cati	Toxascaris leonina	Hookworm	Aelurostrongylus abstrusus	Dipylidium species	Taenia taeniaeformis	Presentation
Piperazine*	Various	Various	+	+	(+)				Tablet
Dichlorophen*	Various	Various						+	Tablet
Praziquantel	Droncit	Bayer					+	+	Tablet/injection
Fenbendazole	Panacur	Hoechst	+	+	+	+		+	Suspension/granules
Mebendazole	Telmin KH	Janssen	+	+				+	Tablet
Pyrantel/Praziquantel	Drontal Cat	Bayer	+	+	+		+	+	Tablet

* Present in some GSL multiwormer products.
+, Claim present on some preparations.

WORM CONTROL

There is a dearth of good information on which to base advice on worm control in cats, particularly kittens. However, based on knowledge of the life cycle of *T. cati*, kittens should be wormed at 5 weeks of age and the treatment repeated at intervals until 12 weeks of age, using an anthelmintic that is effective against *T. cati*. Information derived from puppies infected with *T. canis* would suggest that appropriate retreatment intervals may vary according to the efficacy of the anthelmintic being used. For example, retreatment with fenbendazole, which is likely to be effective against immature *T. cati*, may be required less frequently than retreatment with piperazine which is less likely to be effective against the immature worms.

Adolescent and adult cats should be wormed at 3–6-month intervals using products that are effective against *Dipylidium* species, *Taenia* species and ascarid infection. Choice of the interval recommended and product will be dictated by knowledge of the likely degree of exposure to parasite infection. A combination anthelmintic (Drontal Cat, Bayer has now been introduced. This has a broad spectrum of activity against the common helminth infections of the cat.

Anyone familiar with the anthelmintics available for use in the dog will realize that there are fewer products on the market for use in the cat. This may be because insufficient work has been done to establish safety and efficacy in the cat or because the product is known to be unsuitable for this species. It cannot be assumed that the pharmacokinetics, and hence the dose rate, will necessarily be the same in the dog and cat. It is therefore worthwhile checking with the manufacturer if, for any reason, it is deemed necessary to use a product not recommended for use in the cat.

REFERENCES AND FURTHER READING

Anonymous (1977) Parasites in dogs and cats. *British Medical Journal* **2**, 901.
Anonymous (1985) Answers to your questions about Droncit. *Veterinary Medicine* July 1985 (Suppl.) **80**, 39–42.
Blowers, A. J. (1977) Toxocariasis in perspective. *Royal Society of Health Journal* **97**, 279–280.

Cowper, S. G. (1977) Helminth parasites of dogs and cats and Toxoplasmosis antibodies of cats in Swansea, South Wales. *Annals of Tropical Medicine and Parasitology* **72**, 455–459.

Else, R. W., Bagnall, B. G., Pfaff, J. J. G. & Potter, C. (1977) Endo- and ecto-parasites of dogs and cats: A survey from practices in the East Anglian Region, BSAVA. *Journal of Small Animal Practice* **18**, 731–737.

Hamilton, J. M. (1963) *Aelurostrongylus abstrusus* infestation of the cat. *Veterinary Record* **75**, 16, 417–421.

Manger, B. R. & Brewer, M. D. (1989) Epsiprantel, a new tapeworm remedy. Preliminary efficacy studies in dogs and cats. *British Veterinary Journal* **145**, 384–388.

McColm, A. A. & Hutchison, W. M. (1980) The prevalence of intestinal helminths in stray cats in central Scotland. *Journal of Helminthology* **54**, 255–257.

Niak, A. (1972) Prevalence of *Toxocara cati* and other parasites in Liverpool cats. *Veterinary Record* **91**, 534–536.

Nichol, S. (1982) Parasites of domestic and feral cats from the London Area. BSc Thesis.

CHAPTER 9

Nutritional Support of the Anorexic Cat

ANDREW SPARKES

INTRODUCTION

The role of nutrition in the management of many diseases is now widely accepted in veterinary medicine and the advent of commercial veterinary clinical diets has helped in the practical application of this knowledge to our patients. However, one aspect of nutrition that is not widely used in practice is critical-care nutrition, or nutritional support of the anorexic/inappetent patient. Anorexia or inappetence are encountered in many medical and surgical patients, but the problem of inadequate protein and calorie intake is often overlooked while efforts are made to diagnose and/or, treat the underlying disease. The adverse effects of dehydration are well recognized and fluid therapy forms an integral part of the support of many animals but the potentially devastating effects of malnutrition are often forgotten in these same cases.

In normal individuals, the response to food deprivation (starvation) is an adaptive down-regulation of the basal metabolic rate (mediated in part through lower insulin levels leading to a decreased conversion of T_4 to T_3) which results in a decreased caloric requirement (see Fig. 9.1). Initially, fasting results in rapid utilization of hepatic glycogen to maintain

A. H. Sparkes

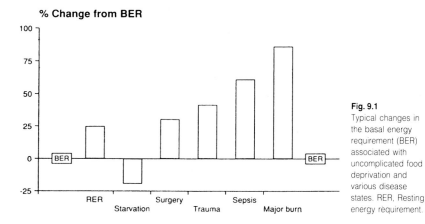

% Change from BER

Fig. 9.1
Typical changes in
the basal energy
requirement (BER)
associated with
uncomplicated food
deprivation and
various disease
states. RER, Resting
energy requirement.

blood glucose levels (glycogenolysis), with considerable depletion of glycogen stores occurring within 24 h. Most body tissues are able to adapt to alternative (non-glucose) sources of energy and, thus, fat from adipose tissue is mobilized by lipolysis, producing free fatty acids and glycerol. Free fatty acids can be used directly by many tissues, and ketones formed from the partial oxidization of fatty acids in the liver are an additional source of energy. The glycerol liberated by lipolysis is utilized by the liver for gluconeogenesis, but this is insufficient to maintain normal blood glucose levels and therefore gluconeogenic amino acids are catabolized to supply adequate glucose to those tissues with an obligatory requirement (e.g. the central nervous system).

THE NEED FOR NUTRITIONAL SUPPORT

In diseased animals, the stress of illness, the processes of tissue repair and immune response, the effects of pyrexia and / or, the demands of neoplastic tissue will affect the normal metabolic response to food deprivation. Generally, there is an increased release of "catabolic" hormones, such as glucagon, catecholamines and cortisol, resulting in abrogation of the adaptive response to decreased food intake and an increase in energy requirements proportional to the severity of the disease process. The increased need for calories and protein in a diseased anorexic/inappetent individual causes an accelerated form of starvation commonly termed protein energy malnutrition (PEM).

The often profound adverse effects of PEM are now well documented. They include: lymphopenia, reduced T-lymphocyte numbers, impaired cell-mediated immune responses, impaired humoral immune response, impaired neutrophil function, reduced serum complement levels, hypoproteinaemia, anaemia, delayed wound healing, delayed fracture healing, muscle weakness, increased incidence of sepsis and increased mortality.

The occurrence and importance of these adverse effects will vary between individuals according to the severity and duration of the PEM and the underlying cause(s) of the malnutrition. However, even moderate malnutrition contributes significantly to increased morbidity and mortality rates which can be reversed by administering nutritional support.

SELECTION OF PATIENTS

Not all inappetent patients require nutritional support but, if appropriate support is to be given, patients either with or at risk of developing PEM must be identified and managed early during the course of the disease to minimize the potentially serious adverse effects.

Identification of these patients is not easy because PEM may have an insidious onset and is not characterized by any specific clinical signs. Ideally, one or more laboratory tests would be used as sensitive and specific markers of PEM to assess objectively nutritional status. But no simple reliable markers are available either in human or veterinary medicine at present; although abnormal results of laboratory tests are often encountered in PEM (e.g. lymphopenia, reduced plasma proteins – albumin, transferrin pre-albumin, etc. – anaemia), they are neither sensitive nor specific indicators. More emphasis has to be placed on various subjective criteria to assess our patients. Guidelines indicating the type of patient that may require support are:

(1) Loss of ≥10% body weight during the preceding 7–14 days

(2) Anorexia or marked inappetence of ≥3 days' duration
(3) Cachexia
(4) Inadequate body fat or muscle mass
(5) Patients with conditions resulting in direct protein/energy loss (e.g. exudative peritonitis/pleuritis, especially when being drained).

Cats presented with any of these signs should have their dietary intake monitored very closely and, if caloric requirements are not being met (see Table 9.3), nutritional support should be instigated immediately.

METHODS OF PROVIDING SUPPORT

There are a variety of methods of providing nutritional support, but two general principles apply: first, whenever the gastrointestinal tract is functional it should be used and, second, the simplest suitable method of providing food should be chosen. Total parenteral nutrition is expensive and technically more difficult to administer than enteral nutrition, and there are relatively few patients that require it. Table 9.1 outlines the common forms of enteral nutritional support available for veterinary patients (references are supplied for techniques not covered in this article).

Table 9.1 Forms of enteral nutritional support.

(1) Appetite stimulation
(2) Force feeding*
(3) Enteral tube feeding   Orogastric*
                                    Nasogastric/nasoesophageal
                                    Pharyngostomy*
                                    Oesophagostomy
                                    Gastrostomy (Lewis *et al.*, 1987, Bright and Burrows, 1988; Crowe, 1989)
                                    Enterostomy (jejunostomy) (Orton, 1986; Crowe, 1989)
(4) Total parenteral nutrition (Lippert and Armstrong, 1990; Lewis *et al.*, 1987).

---

* Not suitable or inadvisable in cats.

APPETITE STIMULATION

With cases of mild to moderate inappetence, if there is no physical impediment to prehension and ingestion of food and if
circumstances allow, attempts at appetite stimulation may be
appropriate. A number of factors which may increase the palatability of food or the desire to eat are:

(1)   Feed the normal home diet – cats often develop strong
preferences linked to familiarity
(2)   Provide wide, shallow food bowls (no interference with
whiskers)
(3)   Offer small amounts of fresh food frequently
(4)   Feed moist rather than semi-moist or dry food
(5)   Feed warm food (80°–100°F)
(6)   Feed a high fat, high protein diet (see Table 9.4)
(7)   Feed foods with strong odours (especially meat, fish or
cheese)
(8)   Provide a comfortable, quiet environment
(9)   Provide physical encouragement (petting and stroking)
(10)   Clean encrustations from the nose, if present
(11)   Provide adequate analgesia if pain is present.

In addition to manipulating the diet, pharmacological stimulation of the appetite may also be employed; some of the agents
available are shown in Table 9.2. The side-effects associated

Table 9.2 Pharmacological stimulation of appetite.

Drug	Route	Dose	Frequency
Diazepam	iv	0.05–0.2 mg/kg	bid/tid
	po	1–2 mg/cat	bid/tid
Oxazepam	po	0.25–0.5 mg/kg	bid/tid
Flurazepam	po	0.1–0.2 mg/kg	bid/tid
Prednisolone	po/im	0.25–0.5 mg/kg	sid
Megestrol acetate	po	1 mg/kg	sid
Stanozolol	po	1–1.25 mg	sid/bid
Nandrolone decanoate	im	5 mg/kg	weekly

iv, intravenously; im, intramuscularly; po, by mouth; sid, once daily; bid, twice daily;
tid, three times daily.

with glucocorticoids and progestogens generally preclude their use as specific appetite stimulants, while anabolic steroids are not as potent as other agents and are of little value in the short-term management of anorexia. Benzodiazepines are effective appetite stimulants in most cats, which probably act by direct appetite stimulation within the central nervous system; individual drugs are not equipotent, their relative activity being structure-dependent. Diazepam is the most widely used drug in this class. It is more effective given intravenously than either intramuscularly or orally, and may be administered up to two or three times daily. As with all benzodiazepines, the dose needed to induce eating will frequently result in sedation and ataxia. Furthermore, in some cats the response to benzodiazepines is poor (especially sick cats), and the appetite stimulant properties frequently decline with continual use. It is generally recommended, therefore, that benzodiazepines are not used for longer than 2 or 3 days.

Other appetite stimulants used in cats include cyproheptadine (which is not recommended as it causes excitation in a proportion of individuals) and B-group vitamins (Macy and Ralston, 1990). The requirement for some B vitamins (niacin and pyridoxine) is approximately four times higher in cats than dogs, and experimental depletion of B vitamins does lead to anorexia. It is important, therefore, to ensure adequate intake of B vitamins (orally or parenterally), although there is little evidence that supplementation of these alone is adequate to overcome clinical anorexia.

Whenever appetite stimulation is employed, it is essential to evaluate critically the success of the therapy. As with the monitoring of any patient at risk of PEM, caloric requirements must be calculated (see Table 9.3), and the weight of food to be consumed over 24 h can be determined once the caloric density of the food is known (Tables 9.4 and 9.5). If caloric intake is inadequate, then other means of providing nutrition, such as enteral tube feeding, should be used.

TUBE FEEDING

A number of different methods are available for tube feeding cats. The simplest are the nasoesophageal and oesophagostomy routes which will be discussed in more detail. Although

Table 9.3 Calculation of protein and caloric requirements.

(1) Calculate basal energy requirement (BER)
    BER (kcal/day) = 30 × body weight (kg) + 70 for cats >2 kg body weight
    BER (kcal/day) = 70 (body weight (kg)$^{0.75}$) for cats of any body weight

(2) Estimate maintenance energy requirement (MER)
    Because of the variable demands of the disease process, in addition to considerable individual variations, it is not possible to determine precisely the MER for each sick cat. However, the BER can be multiplied by the following "stress factors" to arrive at a reasonable approximation of caloric needs.

Disease	Stress factor	Examples
Mild	1.25	Hospitalized sick cat, non-surgical, no infection
Moderate	1.5	Trauma, surgical intervention, mild sepsis/infection, advanced neoplasia
Severe	1.75–2.0	Major surgery, severe infection or sepsis (e.g. peritonitis), head trauma, severe burns

(3) Calculate volume of feed
    Divide MER by the caloric density of the diet (see Tables 9.4 and 9.5) to obtain volume/weight of feed to be given per 24 h

(4) Add a protein supplement if required (see Table 9.5)
    Cats generally require 6–8 g of protein/100 kcal. The levels may need to be adjusted for diseases where protein restriction is desirable or where protein losses are heavy. ProMod (Ross Laboratories) contains 5 g protein per 6.6 g scoop, thus the addition of one scoop to 250 ml of diet containing 1 kcal/ml will increase the protein content by 2 g/100 kcal.

Example of a 4 kg cat with "moderate" disease:
BER = (30 × 4) + 70 = 190; MER = 190 × 1.5 = 285 kcal/day.

pharyngostomy intubation is an established feeding technique, it is associated with a high prevalence of complications, including gagging, airway obstruction and intolerance of the tube. Using a small-bore tube (e.g. 5 FG), and exiting the tube behind the hyoid apparatus in a dorsal position close to the origin of the oesophagus, will help (Crowe and Downs, 1986; Crowe, 1989, 1990), but complications may still arise. To overcome these problems, oesophagostomy intubation (see later) was developed, and the technique appears to be very successful in both dogs and cats (Crowe, 1990).

Gastrostomy intubation has been widely used in cats, particularly in the USA. It is an alternative to oesophagostomy

Table 9.4 Caloric density and nutritional profile of typical canned cat foods, and high fat/high protein/high palatability canned foods.

Food	Caloric density (kcal/100 g) as fed	Protein (% dry weight)	Fat (% dry weight)	Carbohydrate (% dry weight)
Whiskas Supermeat	65	51.0	27.0	9.6
KiteKat Supreme	62	46.2	24.0	18.3
Hill's Science Feline Maintenance	134	43.5	24.1	26.2
Hill's Science Feline Growth	155	47.7	35.3	9.2
Whiskas kitten food	85	54.3	27.7	2.8
Liquivite – Feline Liquid Diet	55	43.1	26.9	21.5
Felistar High Protein	89	45.0	32.5	14.5
Whiskas Feline Concentration Diet	119	45.8	37.5	5.8
Hill's Feline c/d diet	141	43.8	29.3	20.3
Hill's Feline p/d diet	155	49.0	31.9	11.5
Hill's Canine/Feline a/d diet	120	45.7	28.7	17.4

Table 9.5 Liquid tube feeding diets.

Product	Caloric density (kcal/ml)	Osmolality (mOsm/kg)	Protein	Fat	Carbohydrate
				(g/100 kcal [% calories])	
Osmolite*	1.0	310	4.2 (17)	3.4 (30)	13.4 (53)
Jevity*¶	1.0	310	4.2 (17)	3.5 (30)	13.4 (53)
Pulmocare*	1.5	490	4.1 (17)	6.1 (55)	7.0 (28)
Reanimyl†	0.90	323	5.9 (25)	5.5 (50)	6.1 (25)
CliniCare Feline‡	0.92	368	7.6 (30)	5.0 (45)	6.2 (25)
RenalCare Feline‡	0.84	260	5.5 (22)	6.3 (57)	5.4 (21)
Whiskas Feline Concentration Instant Diet §	1.24	383	8.8 (37)	5.2 (47)	3.9 (16)
ProMod*			5 g per 6.6 g scoop		

* Ross Laboratories; † Virbac Ltd; ‡ PetAg/Kruuse; § Waltham; ¶ Contains taurine (meets dietary requirement of cat) and soluble fibre.

intubation for medium to long-term nutritional support, and is particularly useful if support has to be provided for several months. It is also valuable in cases where nasoesophageal or oesophagostomy tubes are contraindicated (e.g. oesophageal dysfunction). Although gastrostomy intubation can be performed at laparotomy, percutaneous placement of the tube with the use of an endoscope (percutaneous endoscopic gastrostomy (PEG) intubation) is a much simpler and less invasive procedure.

Jejunostomy intubation can be used when feeding via the oesophagus or stomach is contraindicated.

NASOESOPHAGEAL INTUBATION

Nasoesophageal tubes are very well tolerated by the majority of cats and have the important advantage of requiring no anaesthesia, and often no sedation, for their placement (see Fig. 9.2). They are particularly valuable in providing short-term (1–2 weeks) nutritional support; although they can be used for longer periods, oesophagostomy or gastrostomy tubes are often more practical for these cases. Other techniques must also be used in cases where nasoesophageal tubes are contraindicated, such as in patients with gastric/oesophageal dysfunction or persistent vomiting. The use of small-diameter nasoesophageal tubes does not prevent voluntary intake of food and there is little problem in judging when to remove the tube.

TECHNIQUE FOR TUBE PLACEMENT

A 4–6 FG human paediatric nasogastric tube is used for cats, 6 FG being suitable for most adult cats. Polyurethane tubes are preferable, having a larger internal diameter and causing less tissue reaction if left *in situ* for prolonged periods, but the cheaper PVC tubes are adequate in most situations (see Table 9.6). If the tubes are not damaged they may be disinfected and reused.

(1)   Pre-measure and mark the tube. Measure from the tip of the nose to the ninth rib – this ensures placement of the tip in

(a)

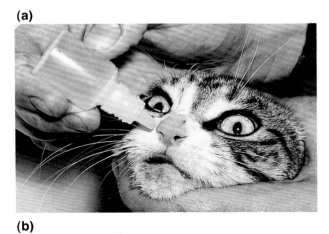

(b)

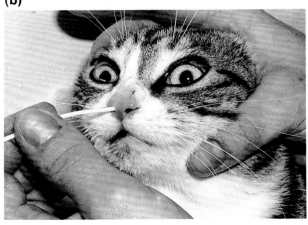

(c)

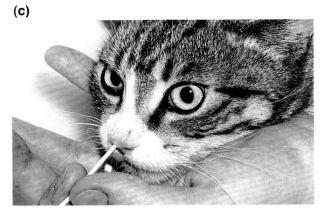

Fig. 9.2
(a) Anaesthetizing the nose. (b) Passing the tube through the nose. (c) Preventing tracheal intubation.

(d)

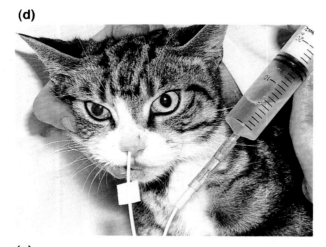

(e)

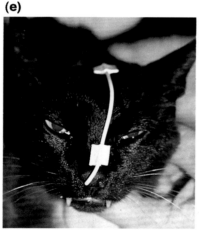

Fig. 9.2
(d) Checking placement. (e) Securing tube. See text for details.

the caudal oesophagus, rather than in the stomach which could lead to reflux oesophagitis and vomiting.

(2)   Anaesthetize the nose. Instil several drops of proxymetacaine hydrochloride (Ophthaine, Ciba-Geigy) (Fig. 9.2a).

(3)   Sedate if necessary. Sedate lightly with, for example, ketamine (Vetalar, Parke Davis), or a ketamine-benzodiazepine combination if necessary.

(4)   Pass the tube through the nose. Lubricate the tube with a water-soluble gel (e.g. KY jelly, Johnson & Johnson) and then pass it into the anaesthetized nose in a ventromedial direction,

Table 9.6 Equipment for tube feeding.

Equipment	Size	Type
Nasogastric tubes		
Corpak Silk Neonata*	5 FG, 56 cm	PU
Corpak Silk Paediatric*	6 FG, 56 cm	PU
XRO Infant Feeding Tube†	4/5/6 FG, 40 cm	PVC
XRO Infant Feeding Tube†	10/12 FG, 50 cm	PVC
Optional equipment‡		
Administration bags and tubes	Flexitainer 500 ml	
	Gavage Sets (gravity drip feeding tubes)	
Administration pumps	Flexiflo I Pump (20–250 ml/h, mains operated)	
	Flexiflo Pump Sets (tubing for pump-assisted administration)	
	Flexiflo Companion Pump (5–300 ml/h, mains/battery operated)	
	Companion Pump Sets (tubing set for Flexiflo Companion Pump)	

PU, Polyurethane, PVC, polyvinylchloride.
* E Merck Ltd; † VygonLtd, ‡ Ross Laboratories.

aiming towards the base of the ear on the opposite side of the head (Fig. 9.2b). The use of a metal guide-wire within the tube is not necessary in cats. If the tube lodges in the dorsal or middle meatus, withdraw it and redirect it ventrally. To prevent tracheal intubation, hold the head in a normal position as the tube approaches the pharynx (Fig. 9.2c).
(5) Check placement of the tube. Inject 5–10 ml of sterile water/saline followed by 5–10 ml of air and auscultate over the left flank. A lack of coughing and audible bubbling sounds (air passing into the stomach) indicate correct placement (Fig. 9.2d). If in doubt, radiography can be used to confirm the position.
(6) Secure the tube. Secure the tube with either:
(i) Sutures: Place a small suture close to the external naris to anchor the tube. Take the tube over the bridge of the nose and attach it to the frontal region with a second suture. This positioning prevents interference with the whiskers which can reduce tolerance of the tube; or
(ii) Superglue: Place small zinc oxide tape "wings" on the tube and then stick them to the hair on the bridge of the nose and the head with Superglue (Fig. 9.2e). Secure the tube to a collar

or neck bandage and fit an Elizabethan collar to prevent tube removal.

CHOICE OF FEEDS

Owing to the narrow diameter of nasoesophageal tubes, only specifically formulated liquid diets (see Table 9.5) can be used in order to avoid tube blockage. In the UK, three veterinary products are currently available – Reanimyl (Virbac), Whiskas Feline Concentration Liquid diet (Waltham), and the CliniCare range (Pet Ag/Kruuse). However, there is a substantial choice of human polymeric (meal replacement) tube diets which may also be used (e.g. Osmolite, Jevity and Pulmocare, Ross Laboratories).

Because the cat has a high dietary protein requirement, most human tube diets need supplementing with a protein additive (e.g. ProMod, Ross Laboratories). Unless protein restriction is indicated, the diet should contain around 6–8 g protein/100 kcal (cf. 4–6 g/100 kcal in dogs). Most human tube diets (with the exception of Jevity) have inadequate levels of taurine for cats, in which it is an essential nutrient; but unless prolonged feeding is undertaken (i.e. more than 4 weeks) this should not cause problems. Arginine is another essential amino acid in cats and deficiency may disrupt the urea cycle resulting in hyperammonaemia and hepatic encephalopathy. Recently, some veterinary and human tube diets have been shown to result in depletion of serum arginine levels and, therefore, some workers routinely add arginine to all tube diets (e.g. 1 mg/kcal) to avoid any potential problems.

The normal osmolality of the small intestinal lumen is around 300–350 mOsm/kg (similar to that of plasma). Isosmolar diets are better tolerated than hyperosmolar diets which either need diluting or a period of gradual acclimatisation for the intestinal tract.

AMOUNT TO FEED

The maintenance energy requirement (MER) is derived from the basal energy requirement plus a "stress factor" (see

Table 9.3). The resultant MER is designed to meet the animal's current requirements and so halt PEM-induced catabolism; generally, restoration of depleted body fat/protein can occur later. Adequate water intake should be ensured – any shortfall may be made up in the form of water or an electrolyte solution (e.g. Lectade, SmithKline Beecham) administered through the nasoesophageal tube.

METHODS OF FEEDING

Feeding can be achieved either by administration of intermittent boluses of food or by continuous drip feeding for prolonged periods.

Regardless of the method of feeding, tube diets ideally should be introduced gradually over 3–4 days. For example:

Day 1: Approximately $\frac{1}{3}$ required amount is fed + $\frac{2}{3}$ water;

Day 2: Approximately $\frac{2}{3}$ required amount is fed + $\frac{1}{3}$ water;

Day 3: The full amount of the tube feed is given.

Bolus feeding

Boluses may be syringed through the nasoesophageal tube at intervals throughout the day. Initially, food should be administered frequently (every 1–2 h) with volumes of up to 20 ml/kg. The amounts and frequency can gradually be adjusted over 2–3 days to meet nutritional requirements. After each feed, the tube should be flushed with water to prevent blockage and plugged to prevent air accumulating in the stomach.

Continuous feeding

Continuous gravity or pump-assisted drip feeding can be conducted throughout the day or for several hours daily. The technique minimizes the risk of diarrhoea (and occasional vomiting) which are mild but not infrequent complications of tube feeding. At regular intervals during feeding (i.e. every 4–6 h) and at the end of feeding, the tube should be flushed and plugged as described above.

If an episode of vomiting occurs, the tube should be checked for correct placement before feeding is recommenced.

COMPLICATIONS

Generally, complications of nasoesophageal tube feeding are rare and usually easily overcome.

Mechanical problems

Occasional individual cats will not tolerate nasoesophageal tubes and another method of feeding must be chosen (e.g. oesophagostomy or gastrostomy). Correct tube placement should always be ensured before feeding commences and, if there is any doubt, radiographic confirmation should be sought. Adequate flushing of the tube with warm water after each feed, followed by plugging, is important to prevent blockage of the tube.

Gastrointestinal problems

Diarrhoea and, less commonly, vomiting occur in a proportion of cases. This is generally a minor complication and can usually be overcome by one or more of the following:

(1)   Using an isosmolar feed rather than a hyperosmolar feed;
(2)   Increasing the frequency and decreasing the volume of bolus feeds;
(3)   Using continuous feeding rather than bolus feeding;
(4)   Reducing the rate of administration;
(5)   Using a higher fat, lower carbohydrate product (see Table 9.5);
(6)   Using a fibre-enriched product (e.g. Jevity).

Metabolic problems

Metabolic problems are rare, but hyperglycaemia and electro-lyte disturbances have occasionally been observed. It is recom-mended that glucose and electrolyte levels should be monitored during the first few days of feeding, and intermittently there-after.

OESOPHAGOSTOMY INTUBATION

Oesophagostomy intubation can be employed where nasoeso-phageal tubes are not tolerated or cannot be used, and is suit-able for longer-term nutritional support (e.g. several weeks). Intubation requires a short, light general anaesthetic. The cat is placed in right lateral recumbency, curved artery forceps are passed into the oesophagus and turned outwards to identify the oesophagus in the left mid-cervical region. The blades of the forceps are opened to allow sharp and blunt dissection from the skin into the oesophageal lumen. The length of tube inserted is calculated as for nasoesophageal tubes and the tip is passed into the oesophagus through the ostomy site. Either a small bore (6 FG) paediatric nasogastric tube can be used, or a larger (10 or 12 FG) tube. The larger tubes may not be as well tolerated by some cats, but they allow administration of a liquidized diet (see Table 9.7). Oesophagostomy tubes should be secured by a Chinese finger-trap suture that also incorporates subcutaneous

Table 9.7 Liquidized diets suitable for tubes ≥10 FG.

Any small-bore tube diet (see Table 9.5)	
Liquivite – Feline Liquid Diet	55 kcal/100 g (see Table 9.4) Strained twice through approximately 1 mm sieve
Home-prepared diet (Crowe, 1989)	½ can (224 g) Hill's Feline p/d 170 ml water 15 ml vegetable (e.g. corn) oil Strained twice through approximately 1 mm sieve

Yields: 120 kcal/100 ml; 7.4% protein; 5.5% fat; 2.8% carbohydrate fascia and skin. Checking tube position, feeding and maintenance is essentially the same as described for nasoesophageal tube feeding.

The complications associated with nasoesophageal tubes may also occur with oesophagostomy tubes. Careful daily cleaning of the ostomy site is essential to prevent secondary infection, and the area should be protected by a neck bandage with the proximal end of the tube secured dorsally. Adequate care of the ostomy site ensures rapid healing by second intention when the tube is removed (Crowe, 1990).

SUMMARY

Over recent years there has been a growing understanding of the impact of malnutrition on the sick patient. The significance of PEM can easily be overlooked, but established techniques readily enable cost-effective nutritional support to be provided. There is no benefit in withholding nutritional support from malnourished inappetent patients. Rather, provision of adequate calories and protein can improve immunocompetence, enhance wound healing, reduce mortality and morbidity rates and improve the quality of life for our patients. The techniques outlined in this chapter, with some minor modifications, are equally applicable to dogs.

REFERENCES AND FURTHER READING

Armstrong, P. J. & Lippert, A. C. (1988) Selected aspects of enteral and parenteral nutritional support. *Seminars in Veterinary Medicine and Surgery (Small Animal)* **3** (3), 216–226.

Bright, R. M. & Burrows, C. F. (1988) Percutaneous endoscopic tube gastrostomy in dogs. *American Journal of Veterinary Research* **49**, 629–633.

Crowe, D. T. (1988) Understanding the nutritional needs of critically ill or injured patients. *Veterinary Medicine* **83**, 1224–1249.

Crowe, D. T. (1989) Nutrition in critical patients: Administering the support therapies. *Vetinary Medicine* **84** 152–180.

Crowe, D. T. (1990) Nutritional support for the hospitalized patient: An introduction to tube feeding. *Compendium on Continuing Education for the Practicing Veterinarian* **12**, 1711–1721.

Crowe, D. T. & Downs, M. O. (1986) Pharyngostomy complications in dogs and cats and recommended technical modifications: experimental and clinical investigations. *Journal of the American Animal Hospital Association* **22**, 493–503.

Lewis, L. D., Morris, M. L. & Hand, M. S. (1987) *Small Animal Clinical Nutrition III*. Kansas, Mark Morris Associates.

Lippert, A. C. & Armstrong, P. J. (1990) Parenteral nutritional support. In *Current Veterinary Therapy X*. (ed. Kirk, R. W.), pp. 26–30. Philadelphia, W. B. Saunders.

Macy, D. W. & Ralston, S. L. (1990) Cause and control of decreased appetite. In *Current Veterinary Therapy X* (ed. Kirk, R. W.), pp. 18–24. Philadelphia, W. B. Saunders.

Orton, E. C. (1986) Enteral hyperalimentation administered via needle catheter-jejunostoma as an adjunct to cranial abdominal surgery in dogs and cats. *Journal of the American Veterinary Medical Association* **188**, 1406–1411.

Wheeler, S. L. & McGuire, B. H. (1990) Enteral nutritional support. In *Current Veterinary Therapy X* (ed. Kirk, R. W.), pp. 30–37. Philadelphia, W. B. Saunders.

CHAPTER 10

Feline Hyperthyroidism

CARMEL MOONEY

INTRODUCTION

Feline hyperthyroidism (thyrotoxicosis) is a multisystemic disorder resulting from high circulating concentrations of tri-
iodothyronine (T_3) and/or, thyroxine (T_4). Although reports of
thyroid tumours appeared sporadically in the early veterinary
literature, hyperthyroidism was not recognized as a clinical
problem until 1979.

Hyperthyroidism is now recognized as the most common
endocrine disease of the domestic cat. However, it is still
unclear whether the increased frequency of diagnosis represents
an actual increase in the number of cases or an improved aware-
ness of the condition by veterinary surgeons together with
easier availability of feline thyroid hormone assays.

Benign thyroid tumours affecting one or both thyroid lobes
are the most common cause of feline hyperthyroidism. Bilateral,
rather than unilateral, lobe involvement occurs in approximately 65% of cases but occasionally ectopic or accessory thyroid tissue may be involved. Thyroid carcinoma, the major thyroid tumour of dogs, is a rare cause of hyperthyroidism in the
cat, accounting for only 2% of all cases.

HISTORY AND CLINICAL FINDINGS

Hyperthyroidism is a disease of middle-aged to old cats. The youngest recorded age at onset is 6 years. There is no breed or sex predisposition.

Signs of hyperthyroidism are insidious and progressive (see Fig. 10.1). They vary from mild to severe depending on the duration of the condition, the ability of a body system to cope with the demands imposed by thyroid hormone excess and the presence of concomitant disease affecting other organs. Table 10.1 lists the most common clinical findings recognized in feline hyperthyroidism. Although most affected animals show evidence of dysfunction of a number of systems, occasionally disturbances in one predominate. Thus, the presence or absence of any particular sign neither confirms nor excludes the diagnosis of hyperthyroidism.

Classically, there is a history of weight loss despite an increased and often ravenous appetite, hyperactivity, polyuria/polydipsia, intermittent diarrhoea and vomiting. Frequently, owners consider these signs simply a part of the general "ageing" process and, as the appetite usually remains good, do not

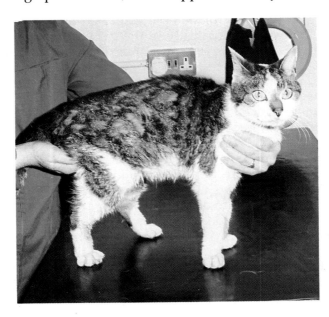

Fig. 10.1
Hyperthyroid, 15-year-old male neutered, domestic shorthaired cat showing poor bodily condition and unkempt coat.

Table 10.1 Major historical and clinical findings in 53 cases of feline hyperthyroidism seen at the Royal (Dick) School of Veterinary Studies.

Finding	Percentage of cats affected
Weight loss	81
Polyphagia	77
Polyuria/polydipsia	70
Tachycardia	64
Diarrhoea (increased frequency, volume, steatorrhoea)	60
Hyperactivity	57
Vomiting	45
Skin lesions (patchy or regional alopecia, mats, harsh dry coat, etc.)	41
Respiratory abnormalities (tachypnoea, dyspnoea, panting, sneezing)	34
Other cardiac abnormalities (powerful apex beat, murmur, gallop rhythm, arrhythmias)	32
Intermittent anorexia	11
Decreased appetite	9
Decreased activity	9
Congestive cardiac failure	7
Palpable goitre	98

seek veterinary attention until the weight loss is severe or the other signs become intolerable.

On examination these cats tend to be restless and aggressive. This behaviour, in conjunction with the disturbances of the cardiovascular system, frequently alert the clinician to the possibility of hyperthyroidism. The latter include tachycardia (heart rate greater than 240 beats/min), murmurs and gallop rhythms. Electrocardiographic changes are common (see Table 10.2) and thoracic radiographs may reveal varying degrees of cardiomegaly. Hyperthyroidism usually induces a form of totally or partially reversible hypertrophic cardiomyopathy, but in some cases this progresses to overt congestive heart failure. Pleural effusion, pulmonary oedema or both will then be evident.

The most specific clinical finding is palpable enlargement of one or both thyroid lobes. Enlargement is detectable by careful palpation on either side of the trachea from the larynx to the thoracic inlet. Affected thyroid glands are freely mobile and may become retrotracheal or, occasionally, intrathoracic. Intra-

Table 10.2 Electrocardiographic changes in 131 cats with hyperthyroidism.

Change	Percentage of cats affected
Tachycardia	66
Increased R wave amplitude	29
Prolonged ORS duration	18
Short Q-T interval	10
Atrial premature complexes	7
Left anterior fascicular block	6
Ventricular premature complexes	2
Right bundle branch block	2
First degree A-V block	2
Second degree A-V block (with ventricular escape complexes)	2
Atrial tachycardia	1
Ventricular tachycardia and bigeminy	1
Ventricular pre-excitation	1

thoracic masses may move cranially if the animal's hindlimbs are gently elevated. The thyroid glands of healthy cats are not palpable.

A form of the disease comparable to apathetic (masked) hyperthyroidism of man occurs in approximately 10% of hyperthyroid cats. These animals are depressed, weak, inappetent or anorexic rather than hyperactive and polyphagic. Accompanying severe cardiac abnormalities (arrhythmias, congestive cardiac failure) or non-thyroidal disorders are common.

The differential diagnoses to be considered for feline hyperthyroidism are chronic renal failure, alimentary lymphosarcoma, diabetes mellitus, idiopathic cardiomyopathy, liver disease and exocrine pancreatic insufficiency.

DIAGNOSIS

LABORATORY FINDINGS

Approximately 15% of affected cats show a mild to moderate erythrocytosis, probably because of a direct effect of thyroid hormones on erythroid marrow and increased production of erythropoietin. Mature leucocytosis and eosinopenia are common, reflecting a stress response.

Elevations in one or more of the following enzymes invariably occur: alanine aminotransferase, alkaline phosphatase, aspartate aminotransferase and lactate dehydrogenase. These are helpful but non-specific diagnostic findings and return to normal with successful treatment.

An increase in the serum thyroid hormone concentrations above the normal range is diagnostic for hyperthyroidism. However, some cats have an elevated T_4 concentration but a normal T_3 concentration. Some of these cats have only mild signs of hyperthyroidism and it is likely that the T_3 concentration would increase into the thyrotoxic range if the condition were allowed to progress untreated. However, severe non-thyroidal illness may also affect the total serum thyroid hormone concentrations. A euthyroid cat with severe non-thyroidal illness would be expected to have T_4 and T_3 concentrations in the low normal or subnormal range. Concomitant hyperthyroidism should therefore be suspected in a cat suffering from non-thyroidal illness where the T_4 and T_3 are high normal or only marginally elevated. On recovery from the non-thyroid illness the thyroid hormone concentrations would increase into the diagnostic range.

THYROID IMAGING

Thyroid imaging using radioactive iodine (^{131}I and ^{123}I) or technetium-99m as pertechnetate ($^{99m}TcO_4$) is a useful diagnostic tool, when available. This technique determines whether there is unilateral or bilateral gland involvement and therefore whether the cat requires unilateral or bilateral thyroidectomy (Fig. 10.2). This is important as in up to 15% of bilateral cases, one thyroid lobe may appear grossly normal at the time of surgery. The technique also determines any alterations in the position of the thyroid glands, the site of hyperfunctioning accessory/ectopic thyroid tissue and the presence of regional or distant metastases from a functioning thyroid carcinoma. However, special facilities are required for this technique and it is usually limited to referral centres.

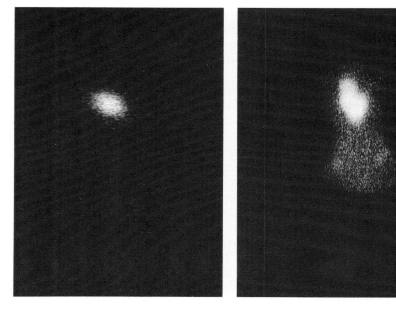

Fig. 10.2 Left: Thyroid scan of a hyperthyroid, 14-year-old, neutered male, domestic shorthaired cat with unilateral (right-sided) thyroid adenomatous hyperplasia. The uninvolved left thyroid cannot be visualized. Right: Thyroid scan of a hyperthyroid 14-year-old, neutered female, domestic shorthaired cat with bilateral adenomatous hyperplasia.

TREATMENT

Surgical thyroidectomy is the most practical treatment for thyrotoxic cats. The best results are achieved when the thyrotoxicosis is controlled prior to surgery. Propranolol, potassium iodide (KI) or antithyroid drugs have commonly been used in the preoperative control of hyperthyroidism. Propranolol, at a dosage of 2.5–5 mg three times daily for 7–14 days, reduces the tachycardia and hyperexcitability associated with hyperthyroidism prior to surgery. KI is reported to block T_4 and T_3 release by the human thyroid gland and also decreases the vascularity and size of the thyroid glands, making surgery more amenable. However, in the author's experience, KI is ineffective in decreasing circulating T_4 and T_3 concentrations to the normal range and an antithyroid drug is preferred.

Antithyroid drugs act mainly by blocking production of thyroid hormones within the thyroid gland. Propylthiouracil, an antithyroid drug previously recommended for use in the cat, has been associated with the production of serious immune-mediated reactions and should no longer be used. Methimazole is associated with fewer side-effects and at a dosage of 5 mg three times daily achieves euthyroidism in 2–4 weeks. However, methimazole is not available in the UK. Carbimazole (Neo Mercazole, Roche) is an alternative, and because it is totally metabolized to methimazole, is used at the same dose rate, achieving euthyroidism in most cats in 2 weeks.

The surgical approach to the feline thyroid gland has been described in detail by Black and Peterson (1983). With the cat in dorsal recumbency and the neck slightly hyperextended, a ventral midline incision is made from the larynx to the manubrium. The sternohyoideus and sternothyroideus muscles are separated by blunt dissection in the midline and retracted to reveal the thyroid lobes (Fig. 10.3). Where thyroid imaging facilities are not available, it is necessary to examine both lobes at the time of surgery to assess whether a unilateral or a bilateral thyroidectomy is required. In those bilateral cases where one lobe appears normal and is not removed, recurrence of the disease usually occurs within 9 months. A biopsy of the apparently normal lobe may indicate the need for future thyroidectomy. The technique for thyroid biopsy involves ligation of the caudal vein, followed by removal of the caudal pole of the gland. Alternatively, a small wedge of tissue may be removed from the caudal pole of the gland.

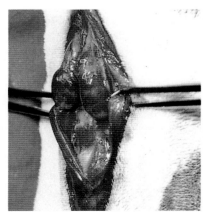

Fig. 10.3
Appearance of affected thyroid gland at the time of surgery.

Prior to thyroidectomy, the external (cranial) parathyroid gland located at the cranial pole of each thyroid lobe, must be identified and at least one preserved to maintain normal plasma calcium concentrations. The internal (caudal) parathyroids are within the body of each thyroid lobe and cannot be preserved. Care must also be taken to visualize and avoid the recurrent laryngeal nerves.

Two techniques have been described for the removal of thyroid lobes. The intracapsular technique, where the thyroid capsule is opened and the gland stripped away leaving the capsule *in situ*, may decrease the incidence of postoperative hypocalcaemia but increases the risk of recurrence because of thyroid tissue adhering to the capsule. The author prefers the extracapsular technique where the thyroid lobe is removed within its capsule and the external parathyroid gland is left *in situ*.

The most important postoperative complication is hypoparathyroidism, which may result if the parathyroid glands are injured, devascularized or inadvertently removed during the course of bilateral thyroidectomy. This results in hypocalcaemia which can manifest as muscle tremors, tetany and generalized convulsions. In the absence of clinical signs, laboratory evidence of hypocalcaemia alone does not warrant treatment, as a low plasma calcium concentration is probably the best stimulus for residual or accessory parathyroid tissue. However, once clinical signs are evident it is necessary to institute prompt therapy (see Table 10.3).

Although hypoparathyroidism can be permanent, spontaneous recovery of parathyroid function can occur weeks to months after surgery either due to recovery of parathyroid tissue temporarily affected by surgery or compensation by accessory tissue. Excising the thyroid lobes in two stages, 3 weeks apart has recently been advocated (Flanders *et al.*, 1987) but, although it decreases the risk of postoperative hypocalcaemia after extracapsular removal of the thyroid glands, it increases the total anaesthetic risk and the cost to the client. Horner's syndrome and voice changes are less common postoperative sequelae.

Table 10.3 Treatment of postoperative hypocalcaemia.

Administer 1–1.5 ml/kg of
   10% calcium gluconate (calcium gluconate injection BP)
or
   10% calcium glubionate (Calcium Sandoz Ampoules 10%, Sandoz)
      slowly intravenously (iv)
      Stop if bradycardia develops

Administer 2 ml/kg of the same solution iv in 120 ml isotonic saline
over the next 12 h. Repeat if required

Begin oral medication as soon as it can be tolerated using
   500–700 mg/kg.day calcium gluconate (calcium gluconate tablets
      BP)
      in three or four divided doses
or
   400–600 mg/kg.day calcium lactate (calcium lactate tablets BP in
      three or four doses)
and
   0.03 mg/kg dihydrotachysterol (AT 10, Sterling Research (solution))
      once daily

Once the plasma calcium concentration is stable, decrease the
dihydrotachysterol by 0.01 mg/kg every alternate day.
Subsequently, assess calcium and dihydrotachysterol requirement
according to plasma calcium concentration.

MEDICAL MANAGEMENT

This form of therapy is recommended for the management of
feline hyperthyroidism where unrelated medical conditions
such as renal failure increase the surgical risk or where owners
refuse surgical treatment. When euthyroidism has been restored
with carbimazole at a dose of 5 mg three times daily, a dose of
5 mg twice daily is usually sufficient for maintenance. Thyroid
hormone concentrations must be regularly monitored and dose
adjustments made if necessary. However, medical therapy is
not without problems. Transient vomiting occurs in approximately 10% of patients but usually does not warrant withdrawal of the drug. Although we have noticed no severe
adverse reactions there remains the possibility that, as with
methimazole, some patients may develop a granulocytopenia
and thrombocytopenia which is reported to occur between
weeks 2 and 12 of therapy. It is therefore recommended that a

Table 10.4 Approach to the hyperthyroid cat.

Confirm diagnosis by T_4 estimation. Assess for any concomitant abnormality, e.g. renal disease	
Surgery	Preoperative treatment with carbimazole (CBZ) 5 mg three times daily until euthyroid Monitor calcium concentrations daily for 3–5 days postoperatively if bilateral Treat if necessary Routinely check for recurrence of hyperthyroidism every 3–6 months
Long-term medical management	CBZ (5 mg three times daily) until euthyroid Maintenance dose of 5 mg twice daily Routinely monitor T_4 concentrations every 6–12 weeks Adjust dose of CBZ if necessary Complete blood count every 2 weeks for first 3 months and monthly thereafter Discontinue therapy if side-effects are noted

complete blood and platelet count be taken every 2 weeks for the first 3 months and monthly thereafter and therapy discontinued as soon as any abnormality is detected. Poor owner compliance in regularly administering the drug is a common reason for failure of therapy. If this is a problem, the drug can be given as a once-daily dose, although this is likely to result in less effective control. A summary of the surgical and medical management of feline hyperthyroidism is given in Table 10.4.

RADIOACTIVE IODINE THERAPY

Radioactive iodine is a simple, safe and effective method of therapy for hyperthyroidism and is considered the treatment of choice for most cats. Radioactive iodine is concentrated within the thyroid gland and selectively irradiates and destroys functional thyroid tissue without damaging associated parathyroid tissue. The lack of suitable facilities for this type of treatment severely limits its usefulness in veterinary practice but it is available in selected referral practices.

ACKNOWLEDGEMENTS

The author would like to thank Dr K. L. Thoday for his special interest and useful comments in preparing this article.

REFERENCES AND FURTHER READING

Black, A. P. & Peterson, M. E. (1983) Thyroid biopsy and thyroidectomy. In *Current Techniques in Small Animal Surgery*, 2nd edn (ed. Bojrab, M. J.), pp. 388–396. Philadelphia, Lea and Febiger.

Flanders, J. A., Harvey, H. J. & Erb, N. (1987) Feline thyroidectomy, a comparison of postoperative hypocalcaemia associated with three surgical techniques. *Veterinary Surgery* **16**, 362–366.

Mooney, C. T. (1994) Radioactive iodine therapy for feline hyperthyroidism. Efficacy and administration routes. *Journal of Small Animal Practice* **35**, 289–294.

Mooney, C. T., Thoday, K. L. & Doxey, D. L. (1992) Carbimazole therapy of feline hyperthyroidism. *Journal of Small Animal Practice* **33**, 228–235.

Peterson, M. E. & Turrel, J. M. (1986) Feline hyperthyroidism. In *Current Veterinary Therapy IX: Small Animal Practice* (ed. Kirk, R. W.), pp. 1026–1033. Philadelphia, W. B. Saunders.

Peterson, M. E., Kintzer, P. P., Cavanagh, P. G., Fox, P. R., Ferguson, D. L., Johnson, G. E. & Becker, D. V. (1983) Feline hyperthyroidism: Pretreatment clinical and laboratory evaluation of 131 cases. *Journal of the American Veterinary Medical Association* **183**, 103–110.

Thoday, K. L. (1988) Feline hyperthyroidism – a review of the literature. In *Advances in Small Animal Practice* (ed. Chandler, E. A.), pp. 120–158. Oxford, Blackwell Science.

Thoday, K. L. & Mooney, C. T. (1992) Historical, clinical and laboratory features of 126 hyperthyroid cats. *Veterinary Record* **131**, 257–264.

CHAPTER 11

Antineoplastic Chemotherapy

RICHARD SQUIRES AND NEIL GORMAN

INTRODUCTION

In recent years, chemotherapy has been used successfully in the treatment of certain small animal tumours. By extrapolation from studies in humans and experimental animals, and partly through trial and error, therapeutic protocols have been devised. It is now possible to treat a variety of tumours with good efficacy and minimal adverse effects. A great deal more is known about canine than feline chemotherapy. The reason for this is purely historical, most investigators having concentrated on the dog rather than the cat. This seems a little unfair, given the increasing popularity of cats as pets and the importance of neoplasia as a cause of illness and death in this species (see Fig. 11.1). Fortunately, a number of recent articles on aspects of feline antitumour chemotherapy have redressed the imbalance somewhat. In general, cats tolerate chemotherapy rather well and their small size makes the use of expensive chemotherapeutic agents far more affordable than it would be in a large dog.

This article is intended to help the clinician to decide if chemotherapy is indicated for a particular feline cancer patient and, if so, to help them institute appropriate therapy and avoid

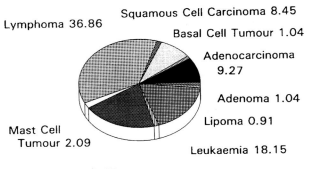

Fibroma 1.26

Squamous Cell Carcinoma 8.45

Lymphoma 36.86

Basal Cell Tumour 1.04

Adenocarcinoma 9.27

Adenoma 1.04

Lipoma 0.91

Mast Cell
Tumour 2.09

Leukaemia 18.15

Others 19.67

Osteosarcoma 1.26

Fig. 11.1
Relative frequencies of
feline tumours (%).

possible pitfalls. Several reviews on the subject of feline oncology and chemotherapy are available (Gorman, 1986; Theilen and Madewell, 1987; Couto, 1989).

OBJECTIVES OF CHEMOTHERAPY

It is rarely possible to cure the feline neoplastic diseases for which chemotherapy is indicated (see Table 11.1). The aim should be to palliate the disease as much as possible while allowing the patient to enjoy a good quality of life. The point about quality of life is an important one. In human medicine,

Table 11.1 Indications for chemotherapy.

Chemotherapy is indicated in a number of circumstances

(1) In patients with systemic, chemosensitive neoplastic disease, such as lymphoma or some leukaemias.

(2) In patients with inoperable, metastatic, chemosensitive neoplasia (for example, metastatic mammary adenocarcinoma).

(3) In patients which have undergone surgery for removal of a tumour with high metastatic potential (postoperative adjuvant chemotherapy).

(4) In situations where complete removal of a malignant chemosensitive tumour is impossible, and radiotherapy is not a viable option.

cancer patients are often treated with high doses of chemotherapeutic agents in an attempt to cure them. These high doses
inevitably produce toxic effects. It is generally accepted that this
approach is unreasonable for pets. This is partly because the
ability to deal with the consequences of toxicity is relatively
poor in small animal practice. The aim should be to achieve as
much as possible while avoiding toxic effects. The poor cure
rate in veterinary chemotherapy is partly a consequence of this
more conservative approach. However, it is frequently possible
to induce complete remission (CR) of the tumour. During CR
the patient should appear and behave as a completely normal
animal. The goal is to prolong CR for as long as possible.
Eventually, the disease will recur and at this stage it is often
resistant to therapy. The options at this stage include intensi-
fication of the chemotherapy, with the attendant risk of toxic
effects, or euthanasia if further chemotherapy is not intended
and the patient is no longer enjoying a good quality of life.

In some patients chemotherapy fails to induce CR. Often
there is a partial remission (PR) and the patient is able to enjoy
life despite persistence of some of the tumour burden. In general, patients which attain only PR have a poorer prognosis than
those reaching CR. Patients that do not respond to chemotherapy (no remission) have the poorest prognosis of all.

INCIDENCE OF NEOPLASIA IN CATS

Although the incidence of neoplasia in cats is approximately
half of that in dogs (MacVean *et al.*, 1978; Priester and McKay,
1980), the percentage of malignant tumours is far higher. In one
study (MacVean *et al.*, 1978) there were 495 tumours per 100 000
cats per year of which 83% were malignant. In the same study
only 35.8% of canine tumours were malignant. The incidence
of various feline tumours is depicted in Fig. 11.1. As can be seen,
lymphoma is by far the most common feline neoplasm compris-
ing 36.86% of all feline tumours. Various forms of leukaemia
contribute a further 18.15%, with squamous cell carcinomas
contributing 8.45%. Adenocarcinomas represent 9.27% of the
total, of which mammary adenocarcinomas contribute 3.44%
and intestinal adenocarcinomas 2.05% of all feline tumours.
Other tumour types occur less frequently.

The predominance of haemolymphatic neoplasms in the cat is in sharp contrast to the dog, in which skin and mammary tumours are the most common types. Feline leukaemia virus (FeLV) is largely responsible for this difference. FeLV is an infectious retrovirus, prevalent among cats, which causes most feline haemolymphatic neoplasms. Approximately 70% of cats with lymphoma and almost all cats with leukaemia have been found to be FeLV-positive (Hardy, 1981a).

PRINCIPLES OF CHEMOTHERAPY

The aim of chemotherapy is to destroy as many tumour cells as possible, while minimizing toxicity to normal tissues. Most chemotherapeutic agents rely on the fact that tumour cells are fast growing and rapidly dividing. Normal tissues are only spared from toxic effects because they are, in general, slower growing. Certain normal cells, such as bone marrow progenitor cells and intestinal epithelium, are very rapidly dividing, indeed they divide faster than many tumours. They are thus highly susceptible to damage by chemotherapy. For this reason most chemotherapeutic drugs have a low therapeutic index (i.e. narrow therapeutic to toxic ratio). Myelosuppression and gastrointestinal signs are common toxic effects of chemotherapy.

Because of the likelihood of toxicity in cases of overdose and the risk of tumour recurrence if the patient is underdosed, it is important that dosing is accurate. For this reason, the more accurate system of dosing according to body surface area (BSA) rather than bodyweight is used by most oncologists. BSA is proportional to metabolic mass and takes into account the higher metabolic rate of smaller animals. Table 11.2 provides a convenient conversion from weight in kilograms (kg) to BSA in metres squared (m^2) for use in cats.

In most circumstances, when treating a tumour it is desirable to use multiple drugs with different mechanisms of action. Greater efficacy and a lower incidence of adverse effects are achieved in this way. Multiple drugs may be given at the same time or in sequence. They are often dosed in a repeating 3- or 4-weekly cycle. Different combinations of drugs and dose intervals (protocols) are used for different tumours. This is because

Table 11.2 Conversion table for weight in kilograms (kg) to body surface area (BSA) in metres squared (m²).

Weight (kg)	BSA (m²)	Weight (kg)	BSA (m²)
2.0	0.159	3.6	0.235
2.2	0.169	3.8	0.244
2.4	0.179	4.0	0.252
2.6	0.189	4.2	0.260
2.8	0.199	4.4	0.269
3.0	0.208	4.6	0.277
3.2	0.217	4.8	0.285
3.4	0.226	5.0	0.292

tumours vary enormously in their sensitivity to chemotherapy. Table 11.3 shows the relative chemosensitivity of a number of common feline tumours.

Chemotherapeutic drugs may be divided into a number of categories, which work by different mechanisms and at different stages in the cell growth cycle:

(1) Alkylating agents cause cross-linking and breaking of DNA molecules, interfering with DNA replication and RNA transcription.
(2) Mitotic spindle inhibitors bind to cytoplasmic microtubular proteins and arrest mitosis in metaphase.
(3) Antimetabolites mimic normal substrates needed for nucleic acid synthesis. They inhibit cellular enzymes or lead to the production of non-functional molecules.

Table 11.3 Relative chemosensitivity of feline tumours.

Highly chemosensitive	Moderately chemosensitive	Chemoresistant
Lymphoma	Mammary adenocarcinoma	SCC
CLL	MCT	Fibrosarcoma
CML	OS	ALL
		AML

CLL, Chronic lymphocytic leukaemia; CML, chronic myelogenous leukaemia; MCT, mast cell tumour; OS, osteosarcoma; SCC, squamous cell carcinoma; ALL, acute lymphoblastic leukaemia; AML, acute myelogenous leukaemia.

(4) Antitumour antibiotics bind to DNA and inhibit DNA and RNA synthesis.

(5) Glucocorticoids are cytolytic for lymphoid tissues and are therefore useful in the treatment of haemolymphatic malignancies. Their mechanism of antitumour action is unclear.

(6) Miscellaneous other agents with a variety of mechanisms of action are used in chemotherapy.

CONSIDERATIONS BEFORE STARTING CHEMOTHERAPY

The administration of chemotherapy is involved, costly and time-consuming for both the client and veterinarian and has the potential to cause serious toxicity to the patient. It should not be undertaken lightly. Before starting chemotherapy, as much as possible should be learned about the neoplastic disease and general health status of the patient. The tumour should not be considered in isolation. There is little point in treating an inoperable oral tumour if the patient is in advanced renal failure. The checklist (below) suggests a database which will enable the clinician to assess the patient thoroughly and offer an informed prognosis to the client.

(1) Thorough physical examination;
(2) Haematology/serum chemistry/urinalysis;
(3) FeLV status;
(4) Chest and abdominal radiographs;
(5) Histological or cytological diagnosis;
(6) Detailed client communication;
(7) ± Informed consent/signature;
(8) ± Bone marrow biopsy;
(9) ± FIV status.

Physical examination, blood work and radiographs will help define the extent of neoplastic disease and may demonstrate other unexpected abnormalities which might influence the prognosis.

FeLV status has a significant effect on prognosis in cancer patients, with FeLV-positive cats generally doing less well. Because FeLV is contagious, FeLV-positive cats undergoing chemotherapy should be kept indoors and denied access to susceptible cats. This restriction may be unacceptable to some clients. Although there is no evidence that FeLV presents a risk to human health, there has been much debate on whether or not FeLV-positive cats should be kept as pets (Hardy, 1981b; Hayes, 1983). Considerations such as these may influence the decision on whether or not to start chemotherapy in an FeLV-positive cat.

At this point it is worth emphasizing that many FeLV-positive cats do not have tumours, and FeLV-positive status is not, in itself, an indication for chemotherapy. Indeed, it is contraindicated unless the cat has a chemosensitive tumour.

A histological or cytological diagnosis is essential if serious mistakes are to be avoided. There are several non-neoplastic lesions of cats which resemble tumours. In most cases a surgical or Tru-cut biopsy of the tumour can be obtained but in some situations, for example mediastinal lymphoma with pleural effusion, a cytological diagnosis obtained by thoracocentesis may suffice. In many cases, chemotherapy can be started on the basis of a cytological diagnosis while waiting for histopathological confirmation.

The importance of careful client communication in anticancer chemotherapy cannot be overemphasized. Once the initial database has been obtained, the clinician should discuss the prognosis for the patient with and without treatment and the likely cost of therapy. Many clients have friends or relatives who have undergone chemotherapy and are frightened about the prospect of "side-effects" in their pet. Although it is important not to underplay the possibility of toxic effects, it is worth pointing out that the doses used in cats are, in real terms, about two or three times lower than those used in human patients. Specifically, cats are most unlikely to become alopecic during treatment, although they may eventually lose their whiskers. The coat will frequently become softer due to the loss of coarse guard hairs. In situations where a client is having difficulty in deciding whether or not to treat a patient because of fears about side-effects a reasonable option is to start treatment and see how the patient responds for 2 or 3 weeks. Often there is a dramatic improvement in the demeanour of the patient and this allays the owner's fears.

Most of the drugs used in feline chemotherapy have not been licensed for use in this species. It is important that the client understands this and gives permission for their use in the patient. Some authorities have suggested that a consent form should be signed by the client (Madewell and Simonson, 1989). The possible toxic effects of chemotherapeutic agents are discussed later.

ANTICANCER CHEMOTHERAPEUTIC AGENTS USEFUL IN CATS

Most of the drugs used to treat cancer are themselves potent mutagens and teratogens. It is wise to take sensible precautions, such as the wearing of disposable gloves, when handling these agents. Table 11.4 summarizes the agents commonly used in feline antitumour therapy.

VINCRISTINE

This mitotic spindle inhibitor is an alkaloid derived from the periwinkle plant (*Vinca rosea* L.). It is a useful part of most chemotherapeutic protocols used in cats. It must be given intravenously and causes severe inflammation and, potentially, necrosis if inadvertently administered perivascularly (see later). Vincristine is moderately myelosuppressive. A rare complication of its use in cats is peripheral neuropathy. Vincristine is fairly expensive. The recommended formulation is a 1 mg/ml aqueous solution which has a good shelf-life.

CYCLOPHOSPHAMIDE

This alkylating agent can be given orally or intravenously. Cyclophosphamide is a pro-drug requiring hepatic activation. It is useful in a wide range of feline neoplasms. Toxic effects seen in some cats are gastrointestinal signs (anorexia, nausea, vomiting) and severe myelosuppression. The sterile cystitis which occurs in dogs and man is less of a problem in cats. The concurrent use of prednisolone in many protocols makes the risk of cystitis even less. Cyclophosphamide is relatively cheap.

Table 11.4 Summary of data on chemotherapeutic agents useful in cats.

Drug	Routes of administration	Dose	Indications	Possible toxic effects
Vincristine	iv	0.5 mg/m² once a week	Many	Local irritant, neuropathy (rare)
Cyclophosphamide	iv, po	50 mg/m² po eod or 100–200 mg/m² iv weekly	Many	Myelosuppression (severe), anorexia
Prednisolone	iv, po, sc	20–40 mg/m² daily to eod	LSA, ALL, CLL, MCT	Few
Doxorubicin	iv	20–30 mg/m² every 3–4 weeks up to 240 mg/m² maximum	Many	Local irritant, myelosuppression (severe), anorexia, nephrotoxicity, cardiotoxicity
Methotrexate	iv, po	2.5–5 mg/m² 2–3 times weekly po or 10–15 mg/m² iv every 1–3 weeks	LSA	Myelosuppression (moderate)
Cytosine arabinoside	iv, sc	100 mg/m² daily for 2 consecutive days (iv infusion)	LSA, AML, ALL	Myelosuppression (severe)
L-Asparaginase	sc, ip	10000 units/m² every 1–3 weeks	LSA, ALL	Possible anaphylaxis
Chlorambucil	po	2 mg/m² eod	LSA, CLL	Myelosuppression (moderate)
Melphalan	po	2 mg/m² eod	CLL, MM	Myelosuppression (moderate)
Hydroxyurea	po	10–50 mg/kg daily to eod	PV, CML	Myelosuppression (severe)

iv, intravenously; po, per os; sc, subcutaneously; ip, intraperitoneally; eod, every other day; LSA, lymphoma; ALL, acute lymphoblastic leukaemia; CLL, chronic lymphocytic leukaemia; MCT, mast cell tumour; PV, polycythaemia rubra vera; AML, acute myelogenous leukaemia; CML, chronic myelogenous leukaemia; MM, multiple myeloma.

PREDNISOLONE

Not often thought of as a chemotherapeutic agent, prednisolone is, nevertheless, cytotoxic for lymphoid tissues and therefore useful in the treatment of lymphoma and some leukaemias. Prednisolone is not myelosuppressive and its side-effects are mostly benign. The doses used in chemotherapy are immuno-suppressive, but most of these patients are, in any case, immunocompromised by their disease. Treatment does not usually make matters worse. Prednisolone penetrates the central nervous system and enters cerebrospinal fluid. Unfortunately, most tumours rapidly become resistant to glucocorticoids.

DOXORUBICIN

This anthracycline antibiotic is a potent, expensive and potentially toxic drug with many uses. It is frequently employed for tumours that are, or have become, resistant to other agents. It is given intravenously. Perivascular injection is calamitous, often resulting in a slough which will not heal. Dilution of the drug 1 : 1 with normal saline and infusion of the solution slowly over 5–10 min through a peripheral venous catheter is recommended. Toxic effects seen in some cats include leucopenia and transient anorexia. Some cats vomit during injection of the drug. Pretreatment with 0.5 mg (total dose) of intravenous dexamethasone (Mauldin *et al.*, 1988) or 0.022 mg/kg of atropine (Jeglum *et al.*, 1985) is reported to reduce the incidence of drug-induced emesis. Serious toxic effects seen after longer-term treatment have been reported. In one study, five cats developed renal disease after cumulative doses of 130–320 mg/m^2 of doxorubicin. Four of these cats showed signs of renal failure (Cotter *et al.*, 1985). In dogs and man, dilated cardiomyopathy is a potential, dose-dependent toxic effect of doxorubicin. Cardiomyopathy has not been reported as a complication of therapy in the cat, but cardiac lesions similar to those found in other species have been found in cats after treatment (Cotter *et al.*, 1985). To reduce the risk of development of cardiomyopathy, it is suggested that a total cumulative dose of 240 mg/m^2 is not exceeded.

METHOTREXATE

This compound inhibits the cellular enzyme dihydrofolate reductase, causing a deficiency of folate coenzymes which are essential for DNA synthesis. The drug can be given orally or intravenously. It is used for the treatment of lymphoma and leukaemia in some practices. Myelosuppression and intestinal epithelial damage are the major toxic effects.

CYTOSINE ARABINOSIDE

This synthetic antimetabolite blocks synthesis of deoxycytidine, a component of DNA. The drug may be given subcutaneously or intravenously (often as a slow infusion over 2 days). It is used in the treatment of lymphoma and some leukaemias. Toxicity is directed at the intestinal epithelium and bone marrow.

L-ASPARAGINASE

This enzyme breaks down extracellular asparagine. Lymphoma cells cannot synthesize this substance and die when it is absent. Normal cells synthesize their own asparagine and are unaffected by the drug. Previously, it was recommended that this agent be given by the intraperitoneal route. Subcutaneous injection is however more convenient and quite satisfactory. L-Asparaginase is a foreign protein, and may provoke an anaphylactic reaction after repeated injections. The clinician should be ready to deal with this complication, should it occur. As with prednisolone, tumours rapidly become resistant to asparaginase. The drug is expensive and has a very short shelf-life once reconstituted. It is available only in aliquots of 10 000 units, enough to treat at least five cats. In some practices, arrangements are made for several patients to be treated with the drug on the same day so that they can share a single vial.

OTHERS

Chlorambucil and melphalan are alkylating agents; both are given orally. Chlorambucil has been used to replace cyclophosphamide in cats which developed the (rare) toxic effect of sterile cystitis during treatment for lymphoma. Melphalan has been used with prednisolone to treat plasma cell neoplasms (Drazner, 1982). Another agent, hydroxyurea, works by inhibiting the enzyme ribonucleoside diphosphate reductase. It is given orally and has been used successfully to treat polycythaemia rubra vera (Couto, 1989).

CHEMOTHERAPEUTIC AGENTS CONTRAINDICATED IN CATS

Cats have gained a reputation for being metabolically incompetent. Perhaps this is because they have difficulty with hepatic glucuronidation of phenolic compounds. Clinically, the most important of these compounds are aspirin and paracetamol. Cats handle many other drugs without difficulty. Indeed, drugs such as aspirin and morphine, once thought to be dangerous in the cat, can be used safely if appropriate dose adjustments are made. Nevertheless, the clinician should recognize that cats are different from dogs and some drugs affect them adversely. Below are two antineoplastic drugs useful in dogs and humans, which are absolutely contraindicated in cats.

(1)   5-Fluorouracil: this antimetabolite causes severe neurotoxicity in the cat, characterized by acute blindness, ataxia and hyperexcitability followed by opisthotonos, convulsions, dyspnoea and death (Harvey et al., 1977; Theilen and Madewell, 1987).
(2)   Cisplatin: this agent, which has a similar mechanism of action to the alkylating agents, is very useful for a wide range of tumours in dogs and man. Unfortunately, even low doses cause pulmonary oedema in the cat as a result of damage to the pulmonary microvasculature. It should not be used in this species (Knapp et al., 1987).

COMPLICATIONS OF CHEMOTHERAPY

PERIVASCULAR INJECTION

If vincristine or doxorubicin are inadvertently injected perivascularly, the needle or catheter should be left in place, and attempts made to withdraw as much of the drug as possible by suction. Once this has been done, the needle is withdrawn, and a 25 gauge needle and syringe are used to withdraw any more of the subcutaneous bleb. Following these measures dexamethasone (0.25 mg/kg) can be injected subcutaneously in the affected area. In cases of doxorubicin leakage, approximately 5 ml of 8.4% sodium bicarbonate can also be injected topically. Application of ice packs to the affected area may be helpful in some cases. Despite these measures, necrosis may occur, producing a lesion like a canine "lick granuloma" or a skin slough. In some cases surgery is necessary.

Clearly, prevention is better than cure. Vincristine and doxorubicin are best administered through a catheter or butterfly needle. It is advisable to dilute these drugs in normal saline for use in cats. This makes the volumes more manageable and reduces the risk of a slough if extravasation occurs. The patient should be well restrained. Before injection of the drug the line should be flushed with normal saline to ensure patency. During injection, patency should be checked frequently by sucking back on the syringe plunger. After injection, the line should be flushed with normal saline before withdrawal of the needle or catheter.

GASTROINTESTINAL SIGNS

Anorexia is the most frequent toxic effect of chemotherapy seen in cats. Cyclophosphamide and doxorubicin often cause this problem. Anorexia may occur immediately after drug administration or a few days later when intestinal epithelial damage is at its height. Anorexia is usually transient and does not limit therapy. Vomiting is a much less frequent problem in cats, although it may occur during injection of doxorubicin (see above). Diarrhoea is a rare complication of chemotherapy in cats.

MYELOSUPPRESSION/SEPSIS

Fast-dividing bone marrow cells are killed by most chemotherapeutic agents. As a consequence, peripheral blood cytopenias
occur, with the lowest point, or nadir, usually 5–10 days after
drug administration. Neutropenia and thrombocytopenia are
the most frequent cytopenias because of the relatively short life
spans of the cells in the peripheral blood (6–8 h for neutrophils
and 5–7 days for platelets). Cell counts usually return to normal
2–3 days after the nadir. Bleeding as a consequence of chemo-
therapy-induced thrombocytopenia is rare, but neutropenia can
cause problems with infections. In a new patient, it is worth
checking a neutrophil count about a week after giving myelosuppressive drugs for the first time. If the neutrophil count is
below 1500 per ml subsequent doses of the agent or agents
responsible should be reduced by 25%. It is prudent to treat
such neutropenic cats prophylactically with a broad-spectrum
oral antibiotic for a few days. A trimethoprim/sulphadiazine
combination is recommended. Any cat which becomes ill after
chemotherapy should have its rectal temperature checked.
Many clients are able to do this at home. If the patient is pyrexic,
a neutrophil count should be obtained. Pyrexic, neutropenic,
sick cats should be assumed to be septicaemic and should be
hospitalized for broad-spectrum, bactericidal antibiotic therapy.
The combination of intravenous gentamicin (1.5 mg/kg every
8 h) and ampicillin (20 mg/kg every 8 h) is useful in this situation. Many of these cats will also require fluid therapy.

CHEMOTHERAPY OF SPECIFIC TUMOURS

LYMPHOMA

The various anatomic forms of feline lymphoma (mediastinal,
alimentary, renal, multicentric and extranodal) have been
reviewed (Couto, 1989). Lymphoma should be regarded as a
systemic disease; in all forms chemotherapy is appropriate,
either alone or as an adjunct to surgery or radiotherapy. Lymphoma is by far the most common feline neoplasm and there
have been several reports on treatment and prognostic factors
(Jeglum et al., 1987; Mooney et al., 1989).

Most cats presented to the veterinarian for lymphoma are ill because of their disease. Without treatment most would be dead within a few weeks, many much earlier than that. In a study of 103 cats treated for lymphoma, 62% attained CR with a median survival time of 7 months; 20% attained PR (median survival time 2.5 months) and 18% had a minimal response (median survival 1.5 months). Approximately one in five cats survived for longer than 1 year. Chemotherapy was judged to be well tolerated by the cats (Mooney *et al.*, 1989).

Several treatment protocols have been described for feline lymphoma. Most use vincristine, cyclophosphamide and prednisolone as the core drugs. When the disease becomes resistant to these drugs, doxorubicin or L-asparaginase are often used in an attempt to re-establish remission. Table 11.5 shows

Table 11.5 Suggested protocol for induction and maintenance therapy in feline lymphoma.

Induction	
Week 1	
Day 1	L-Asparaginase, 10 000 iu/m^2 sc (if available)
	Vincristine, 0.5 mg/m^2 iv
Days 3, 4, 5 and 6	Cyclophosphamide, 50 mg/m^2 po daily
Days 1–7	Prednisolone, 40 mg/m^2 po daily
Weeks 2–8	Vincristine, 0.5 mg/m^2 iv weekly
	Cyclophosphamide, 50 mg/m^2 po eod
	Prednisolone, 20 mg/m^2 po daily
Maintenance	Vincristine, 0.5 mg/m^2 iv fortnightly
	Cyclophosphamide, 50 mg/m^2 po eod*
	Prednisolone, 20 mg/m^2 po eod
Alternative maintenance (not requiring iv drugs)	Chlorambucil, 2 mg/m^2 po eod
	Methotrexate, 2.5 mg/m^2 po 2–3 times weekly
	Prednisolone, 20 mg/m^2 po eod
Treatment of first tumour recurrence	Repeat weeks 2–8 with the prednisolone dose at 40 mg/m^2 rather than 20 mg/m^2
Treatment of subsequent tumour recurrences	L-Asparaginase, 10 000 iu/m^2 sc every 3 weeks until the tumour becomes resistant
	Doxorubicin, 30 mg/m^2 iv every 3 weeks until total cumulative dose reaches 240 mg/m^2

* Chlorambucil, 2 mg/m^2 po eod, can be used to replace cyclophosphamide if sterile cystitis occurs

a protocol for induction and maintenance therapy for feline lymphoma.

LYMPHOID LEUKAEMIA

Diseases in this category include acute lymphoblastic leukaemia (ALL), chronic lymphocyte leukaemia (CLL) and multiple myeloma. Of the three, ALL is the most common and has the most aggressive course. ALL is poorly responsive to chemotherapy. It is important to distinguish ALL from lymphoma with secondary bone marrow involvement because patients in the latter group have a much better prognosis. ALL is treated with the same protocol as that used for lymphoma.

CLL and multiple myeloma are uncommon in the cat. Clinical signs are often vague, and diagnosis is based on peripheral blood or bone marrow findings. Relatively few cats have been treated for these disorders, but a combination of melphalan ($2 \, mg/m^2$ per os every other day) and prednisolone ($20 \, mg/m^2$ per os every other day) has been used with success in both diseases (Couto, 1989).

MYELOID LEUKAEMIA

The term myeloid leukaemia refers to neoplasms arising from any of the cell lines in bone marrow except lymphoid cells. Most cats with myeloid leukaemia are FeLV-positive. There are many types of myeloid leukaemia, which are often difficult to distinguish clinically. There are few reports of successful treatment of myeloid leukaemias. This is partly because these conditions are fairly uncommon, but mainly because therapy is usually unrewarding.

SQUAMOUS CELL CARCINOMA

Squamous cell carcinomas (SCCs) are common in the cat, especially in sunny parts of the world. The ear pinae, nose and oropharynx are most frequently affected. Often these tumours cannot be completely resected and adjunctive radiation therapy is indicated. In situations where radiotherapy is unavailable or otherwise impracticable, chemotherapy can be used. Chemotherapy is also indicated in the occasional case of widespread metastatic SCC. Unfortunately, SCC is relatively chemoresistant. A protocol using doxorubicin and cyclophosphamide produced little or no response in five cats (Mauldin *et al.*, 1988). Doxorubicin (20–30 mg/m^2 every 3–4 weeks) and bleomycin (10 iu/m^2 for 4 consecutive days and then weekly) was helpful in one of four cats with metastatic SCC (Couto, 1989). Another report describes the use of cis-retinoic acid (a derivative of vitamin A) in the treatment of feline SCC of the head (Evans *et al.*, 1985). Retinoic acids are thought to act by inducing differentiation of neoplastic cells. In this study there was poor efficacy and a high incidence of adverse effects (epiphora, blepharospasm and periocular erythema). On this evidence, cis-retinoic acid cannot be recommended as an appropriate treatment for feline SCC.

MAMMARY ADENOCARCINOMA

After haemolymphatic and skin neoplasms, mammary tumours are the next most common type in the cat. Unlike in the dog, the vast majority of feline mammary tumours are malignant and early metastasis occurs. Surgery is most likely to be curative if it is radical and is carried out as early as possible in the course of the disease. Two studies have demonstrated the value of chemotherapy in treating advanced, inoperable or metastatic mammary adenocarcinoma (Jeglum *et al.*, 1985; Mauldin *et al.*, 1988). Adjuvant chemotherapy after resection of large malignant feline mammary tumours should be undertaken, even if there is no evidence of metastasis. It is recommended that treatment be given for 6 months following tumour resection, although there is no published data to support this recommendation. A recommended protocol is as follows:

Day 1:   Doxorubicin 25 mg/m^2 iv.

Days 3, 4, 5, 6: Cyclophosphamide 50 mg/m^2
                  po daily.

Day 10:   Neutrophil count. If count is <1500/ml, give
                  prophylactic oral trimethroprim/sulpha-
                  diazine for 7 days and reduce the dose of

both drugs by 25% next time.

Repeat cycle every 21 days (i.e. day 22 = day 1).

FIBROSARCOMA

Fibrosarcoma in the cat may present as a multicentric or solitary disease. Multicentric fibrosarcoma is a rare condition seen in young cats and is caused by the retrovirus feline sarcoma virus. Multicentric fibrosarcoma has an aggressive, rapidly progressive course. Solitary fibrosarcomas occur more commonly in older cats and are usually found on the limbs, head or neck. They are locally invasive and require radical surgery for total excision. When a limb is affected, amputation may provide the only opportunity for total removal of the tumour. In other situations resection is often complicated by the presence of a pseudocapsule which gives the appearance of a clean margin. This often results in an incomplete primary resection of the tumour mass. If complete resection is impossible, adjuvant radiation or chemotherapy is recommended. Doxorubicin appears to have efficacy when used as a single agent in this disease (Couto, 1989). Other workers have used protocols containing vincristine, cyclophosphamide and methotrexate with variable results.

MAST CELL TUMOUR

Mast cell tumours (MCTs) are uncommon in the cat. In dogs, the vast majority of MCTs are cutaneous. Cats have three main types of MCT: systemic, intestinal and cutaneous. Because the bone marrow is primarily affected in systemic MCT, it may be termed mast cell leukaemia. Optimal therapy for feline MCT is unresolved. In cats with solitary cutaneous or intestinal lesions, wide excision may be curative. In systemic MCT, prednisolone ($40 \, \text{mg/m}^2$ per os daily for 1 week, then $20 \, \text{mg/m}^2$ every other day) is recommended. There is usually splenomegaly in cats with systemic MCT. Splenectomy may be indicated to reduce the tumour burden.

OSTEOSARCOMA

Osteosarcoma (OS) is a rare tumour occurring most commonly in the long bones of older cats. Amputation of the affected limb is the usual therapy. Compared with the dog, the prognosis for feline OS is very good. Cats with appendicular OS have a much better prognosis than those with axial OS (Bitetto *et al.*, 1987). Chemotherapy can be used for inoperable axial disease or for metastases. A protocol using 0.5 mg/m² vincristine, 50 mg/m² cyclophosphamide and 2.5 mg/m² methotrexate given twice monthly for 4 months caused 80% reduction in the size of one ilial OS in a cat. Eight months after the end of the course of chemotherapy the tumour recurred rapidly and was refractory to therapy (Bitetto *et al.*, 1987).

CONCLUSIONS

Although chemotherapy is unable to cure the feline neoplastic diseases for which it is indicated, it can cause temporary disappearance of the tumour and prolongation of good quality life. When chemotherapy is used prudently, the incidence of adverse effects is low. Even if they do occur, adverse effects are often mild and transient. If an individual cat responds poorly to therapy, the option of euthanasia to prevent suffering is always available.

Despite its proven efficacy, few veterinarians in the UK are using chemotherapy in cats. Yet we are quite prepared to treat non-neoplastic diseases, such as dilated cardiomyopathy and advanced chronic renal failure, which have a poorer prognosis with treatment than some neoplastic diseases. Perhaps it is the laudable precept, first do no harm, which inhibits us. Certainly chemotherapy does have the potential to cause harm. Much of this chapter has been devoted to the potential complications of chemotherapy the intention being to forewarn and forearm, rather than to scare the clinician. In fact, the majority of patients receiving chemotherapy have few, if any, problems and are a delight to their owners. Owners are extremely grateful for an alternative to immediate or early euthanasia.

REFERENCES

Bitetto, W. V., Patnaik, A. K., Schrader, S. C. & Mooney, S. C. (1987) Osteosarcoma in cats: 22 cases (1974–1984). *Journal of the American Veterinary Medical Association* **190**, 91–93.

Cotter, S. M., Kanki, P. J. & Simon, M. (1985) Renal disease in five cats treated with adriamycin. *Journal of the American Animal Hospital Association* **21**, 405–409.

Couto, C. G. (1989) Oncology. In *The Cat – Diseases and Clinical Management* (ed. Sherding, R. G.), pp. 589–647. New York, Churchill Livingstone.

Drazner, F. H. (1982) Multiple myeloma in the cat. *Compendium on Continuing Education for the Practicing Veterinarian* **4**, 206–213.

Evans, A. G., Madewell, B. R. & Stannard, A. A. (1985) A trial of 13-cis-retinoic acid for treatment of squamous cell carcinoma and preneoplastic lesions of the head in the cat. *American Journal of Veterinary Research* **46**, 2553–2557.

Gorman, N. T. (1986) Use of cytotoxic drugs in the management of neoplasia. In *Contemporary Issues in Small Animal Practice*, Vol. 6: *Oncology* (ed. Gorman, N. T.), pp. 121–146. New York, Churchill Livingstone.

Hardy, W. D. (1981a) Hematopoietic tumours of cats. *Journal of the American Animal Hospital Association* **17**, 921–940.

Hardy, W. D. (1981b) The feline leukaemia virus. *Journal of the American Animal Hospital Association* **17**, 951–980.

Harvey, H. J., MacEwan, E. G. & Hayes, A. A. (1977) Neurotoxicosis associated with the use of 5-Fluorouracil in five dogs and one cat. *Journal of the American Veterinary Medical Association* **171**, 277–278.

Hayes, A. A. (1983) Care of the feline leukaemia virus positive normal cat. In *Current Veterinary Therapy VIII* (ed. Kirk, R. W.), pp. 411–413. Philadelphia, W. B. Saunders.

Jeglum, K. A., deGuzman, E. & Young, K. M. (1985) Chemotherapy of advanced mammary adenocarcinoma in 14 cats. *Journal of the American Veterinary Medical Association* **187**, 157–160.

Jeglum, K. A., Whereat, A. & Young, K. (1987) Chemotherapy of lymphoma in 75 cats. *Journal of the American Veterinary Medical Association* **190**, 174–178.

Knapp, D. W., Richardson, R. C. & DeNicola, D. B. (1987) Cisplatin toxicity in cats. *Journal of Veterinary Internal Medicine* **1**, 29–32.

MacVean, D. W., Monlux, A. W., Anderson, P. S., Silberg, S. L. & Roszel, J. F. (1978) Frequency of canine and feline tumours in a defined population. *Veterinary Pathology* **15**, 700–715.

Madewell, B. R. & Simonson, E. R. (1989) Special considerations in drug preparation and administration. In *Current Veterinary Therapy X* (ed. Kirk, R. W.), pp. 475–481. Philadelphia, W. B. Saunders.

Mauldin, G. N., Matus, R. E., Patnaik, A. K., Bond, B. R. & Mooney, S. C. (1988) Efficacy and toxicity of doxorubicin and cyclophosphamide used in the treatment of selected malignant tumours in 23 cats. *Journal of Veterinary Internal Medicine* **2**, 60–65.

Mooney, S. C., Hayes, A. A., MacEwan, E. G., Matus, R. E., Geary, A. & Shurgot, B. A. (1989) Treatment and prognostic factors in lymphoma in cats: 103 cases (1977–1981). *Journal of the American Veterinary Medical Association* **194**, 696–699.

Priester, W. A. & McKay, F. W. (1980) The occurrence of tumours in domestic animals. *National Cancer Institute Monograph* **54**.

Theilen, G. H. & Madewell, B. R. (1987) Clinical application of cancer chemotherapy. In *Veterinary Cancer Medicine,* 2nd edn (eds. Theilen, G. H. & Madewell, B. R.), pp. 183–196. Philadelphia, Lea & Febiger.

Index